More Praise for
Elizabeth Wurtzel's
Prozac Nation

"Wurtzel's book is an intelligent, poignant, and unexpectedly witty account of her battle with depression. A beneficiary of modern psychopharmacology herself, she is still able to raise searching questions about the serious issues of medication and emotional illness."
—Barbara Gordon, author of *I'm Dancing as Fast as I Can*

"Wurtzel's memoir of a gifted woman's breakdowns in the fast lane is alternately comedic and wrenching—and always true to life."
—Peter Kramer, M.D., author of *Listening to Prozac*

"Wurtzel is a very entertaining nut case. Reading this book is like being locked up with her, covering your ears or laughing out loud, depending on your perspective. *Prozac Nation* gives a view of every aspect of depression: the self-pity, the courage, the flashes of insight, the despair, and the endless, very moving struggle, simply, to live."
—Jeffrey Eugenides, author of *The Virgin Suicides*

"In punchy, sexy prose, Elizabeth Wurtzel plummets you into the darkness of her innermost experience to emerge once again into medicine, daylight, insight. Abandon whatever you are doing and read this book." —Melanie Thernstrom, author of *The Dead Girl*

"A dangerous book to read. You begin, intending perhaps to get acquainted with the interesting topic of irrational, demonic depression, but after just a few pages, you get the uneasy sensation that the topic is getting acquainted with you."
—Amanda Filipacci, author of *Nude Men*

"A scary glimpse into a private hell. One has to admire her courage for writing her way out. And for questioning the smile-button optimism of the pharmaceutical companies' brave new world."
—Ron Rosenbaum, author of *Travels with Doctor Death*

PROZAC NATION

Young and Depressed in America

✳ ✳ ✳

Elizabeth Wurtzel

RIVERHEAD BOOKS, NEW YORK

Author's Note: Long before Derrida and deconstruction, the Talmud said, quite sagely, "We do not see things as they are. We see them as we are." As far as I am concerned, every word of this book is the complete and total truth. But of course, it's my truth. So to protect the innocent— as well as the guilty—I have changed most names. Otherwise, unfortunately for me, every detail is accurate.

Riverhead Books
Published by The Berkley Publishing Group
200 Madison Avenue
New York, NY 10016

Book design by Rhea Braunstein
Cover illustration © Amy Guip

Houghton Mifflin edition / September 1994
Hardcover ISBN: 0-395-68093-X
Riverhead edition: October 1995
Riverhead ISBN: 1-57322-512-6

Credit lines appear on page 369

Library of Congress Cataloging-in-Publication Data
Wurtzel, Elizabeth.
Prozac nation: young and depressed in America / Elizabeth
Wurtzel.
p.   cm.
Originally published: Boston: Houghton Mifflin, 1994.
ISBN 1-57322-512-6
1. Wurtzel, Elizabeth—Mental health.   2. Depressed persons—
United States—Biography.   I. Title.
RC537.W87   1995
616.[B]85'27'0092—dc20   95—3984   CIP
[B]

For my mom,
lovingly

Very early in my life it was too late.

MARGUERITE DURAS

THE LOVER

Contents

✳ ✳ ✳

PROZAC
NATION

Prologue: I Hate Myself and I Want to Die

* * *

I start to get the feeling that something is really wrong. Like all the drugs put together—the lithium, the Prozac, the desipramine, and Desyrel that I take to sleep at night—can no longer combat whatever it is that was wrong with me in the first place. I feel like a defective model, like I came off the assembly line flat-out fucked and my parents should have taken me back for repairs before the warranty ran out. But that was so long ago.

I start to think there really is no cure for depression, that happiness is an ongoing battle, and I wonder if it isn't one I'll have to fight for as long as I live. I wonder if it's worth it.

I start to feel like I can't maintain the facade any longer, that I may just start to show through. And I wish I knew what was wrong.

Maybe something about how stupid my whole life is. I don't know.

My dreams are polluted with paralysis. I regularly have night visions where my legs, though attached to my body, don't move much.

I try to walk somewhere—to the grocery store or the pharmacy, no-where special, routine errands—and I just can't do it. Can't climb stairs, can't walk on level ground. I am exhausted in the dream and I become more exhausted in my sleep, if that's possible. I wake up tired, amazed that I can even get out of bed. And often I can't. I usually sleep ten hours a night, but often it's many more. I am trapped in my body as I have never been before. I am perpetually zonked.

One night, I even dream that I am in bed, stuck, congealed to the sheets, as if I were an insect that was squashed onto the bottom of someone's shoe. I simply can't get out of bed. I am having a nervous breakdown and I can't move. My mother stands at the side of the bed and insists that I could get up if I really wanted to, and it seems there's no way to make her understand that I literally *can't* move.

I dream that I am in terrible trouble, completely paralyzed, and no one believes me.

In my waking life, I am almost this tired. People say, Maybe it's Epstein-Barr. But I know it's the lithium, the miracle salt that has stabilized my moods but is draining my body.

And I want out of this life on drugs.

I am petrified in my dream and I am petrified in reality because it is as if my dream is reality and I am having a nervous breakdown and I have nowhere to turn. Nowhere. My mother, I sense, has just kind of given up on me, decided that she isn't sure how she raised this, well, this thing, *this rock-and-roll girl who has violated her body with a tattoo and a nose ring, and though she loves me very much, she no longer wants to be the one I run to. My father has never been the one I run to. We last spoke a couple of years ago. I don't even know where he is. And then there are my friends, and they have their own lives. While they like to talk everything through, to analyze and hypothesize, what I really need, what I'm really looking for, is not something I can articulate. It's nonverbal: I need* love. I need the thing that happens when your brain shuts off and your heart turns on.

And I know it's around me somewhere, but I just can't feel it.

What I do feel is the scariness of being an adult, being alone in this big huge loft with so many CDs and plastic bags and magazines and pairs of dirty socks and dirty plates on the floor that I can't even see the floor. I'm sure that I have nowhere to run, that I can't even walk anywhere without tripping and falling way down, and I know I want out of this mess. I want out. No one will ever love me, I will live and die alone, I will go nowhere fast, I will be nothing at all. Nothing will work out. The promise that on the other side of depression lies a beautiful life, one worth surviving suicide for, will have turned out wrong. It will all be a big dupe.

It is Saturday night, we're about at that point when it starts to be Sunday morning, and I am curled up in fetal position on my bathroom floor. The black chiffon of my dress against the stark white tiles must make me look like a dirty puddle. I can't stop crying. The twenty or so people who are still sitting in the living room don't seem at all fazed by what's going on with me in here, if they notice at all, between sips of red wine and hits on a joint someone rolled earlier and chugs on Becks or Rolling Rock. We decided—my house-mate, Jason, and I—to have a party tonight, but I don't think we meant for two hundred people to turn up. Or maybe we did. I don't know. Maybe we're still the nerds we were in high school who get enough of a kick out of the possibility of being popular that we actually did bring this on ourselves.

I don't know.

Everything seems to have gone wrong. First, Jason opened the fire escape door even though it was the middle of January because it had gotten so hot with the crush of bodies, and my cat decided to make the six-flight climb down into the courtyard, where he got lost and confused and started howling like crazy. I didn't have any shoes on and I was worried for him, so I ran down barefoot and it was freezing and it really shook me up to come back in to so many people I had to say, *Hello, how are you?* to, people who didn't know I have a cat that I am absolutely crazy about. For a while Zap and I hid in my room. He curled up on my pillow and gave me a look like all this was my fault. Then my friend Jethro, seeing that I was scared of all these people, offered to do a run up to 168th Street and get some cocaine, which would maybe put me in a better mood.

Being on so many psychoactive drugs, I don't really mess with recreational controlled substances. But when Jethro offered to get me something that might possibly alter my state just enough so I wouldn't want to hide under the covers, I thought, Sure, why not?

There's more: Part of the reason I am so meek is that I stopped taking my lithium a few weeks before. It's not that I have a death wish, and it's not that I'm like Axl Rose and think that lithium makes me less manly (he supposedly stopped taking it after his first wife told him that his dick wasn't as hard as it used to be and that sex with him was lousy; not having that kind of equipment, I'm in no position to give a shit). But I had my blood levels taken at the laboratory about a month ago, and I had an unusually high concentration of thyroid stimulating hormone (TSH)—about ten times the normal amount—which means that the lithium is wreaking havoc on my glands, which means that I could end up in a really bad physical state. Graves' disease, which is a hyperthyroid condition, runs in my family, and the treatment for it makes you fat, gives you these bulging, ghoulish eyes and creates all kinds of symptoms that I think would make me more depressed than I am without lithium. So I stopped taking it. The psychopharmacologist (I like to call his office the Fifth Avenue Crack House, because all he really does is write prescriptions and hand out pills) told me I shouldn't. He told me that, if anything, the lithium was going to give me a condition the opposite of Graves' disease ("What does that mean?" I asked. "Will my eyes shrink up like crinkly little raisins?"), but I don't trust him. He's the pusherman, and it's in his interest to see that I stay loaded.

But he was right. Off lithium, I was fading fast. Some days, I'd sit with Jason reading the *Times* in the living room and I'd talk a blue streak, presenting him with all my theories about, say, the deterioration of the American family in the late twentieth century and how it all relates to the decline of an agrarian society. And Jason would mostly sit there, absorbed in the paper, wondering if I would ever shut up. But then most days I'd be bummed out, plain and simple, ineffectual, going blank again.

I really needed my lithium. But I was determined to cold-kick it. If cocaine would help, so be it. Coke may be really bad for you in every possible way, but it wouldn't give me a thyroid disease, thereby turning me into a younger version of my hysterical, exhausted, overwrought mother. So I did a few lines in the bathroom with Jethro, cutting them up on a Pogues CD. Not five minutes after the stuff first started floating around in my brain, I felt a whole lot better. I went out and mixed and mingled. I walked up to strangers and asked if they were having fun. When new guests arrived, I greeted them, kissing them on each cheek, European-style. I offered to fetch a beer or mix a screwdriver, give them a tour of the apartment, or show them where they should throw their coats. I said things like: There's someone you simply *must* meet. Or, grabbing some girl's hand and pulling her across the room: Have I got the guy for *you*. I was magnanimous and gregarious and all that stuff.

And then, a couple of hours later, I started coming down. I don't drink, so I didn't have any alcohol in my system to

take the edge off what was happening. But suddenly, everything turned ugly, grotesque. Spooky holograms all over the
walls, like acid flashbacks without the color or wonder or
other redeeming features. I felt a panic, as if there were things
I needed to do while I was still on a coke high, and I had
better do them before I completely dropped off. There was
the guy I spent a misbegotten night with who said he'd call
me and never did but came to the party anyway, and I felt
primed for a confrontation. There was my dad, who I really
wanted to call just then, if only to remind him that he still
owed me my allowance from the four years in high school
when I couldn't find him. There were a zillion other things
to do, but I couldn't remember what they were. I knew only
that I wanted a few more minutes to live in this charmed,
enchanted, wired state. I wanted just a little more time to feel
free and easy and unhampered before returning to my depression. I wanted more coke. MORE! COKE! NOW! I
started looking around the bathroom to see if there were any
little bits of the powder left so I could keep it going.

As I patted my hands around the sink and frisked the
floor, I got the weird sense that this sort of behavior maybe
had its place in the eighties, but it seemed really stupid right
now, completely passé in the ascetic, adult nineties. And then
I reminded myself that life is not a media-generated trend, I'll
be damned if I'm going to deny myself just because of Len
Bias and Richard Pryor and whoever else.

So I'm getting ready to ask Jethro to go back up to Spanish Harlem to get us some more of this stuff. I'm making plans,
I'm thinking grandiose thoughts, I'm listing all the people I'm
going to call once I'm coked up again and have the nerve.
I'm deciding to spend the whole night writing an epic
Marxist-feminist study of Biblical villainesses which I've been
meaning to get started on for years. Or maybe I'll just find a
twenty-four-hour bookstore and get a copy of *Gray's Anat-*

omy and memorize it in the next few hours, apply to medical school, and become a doctor and solve all my problems and everyone else's too. I've got it all worked out: *Everything is going to be just fine.*

But before any of this can happen, I crumple onto my bed and start to weep uncontrollably.

Christine, my best friend, comes in to ask what's wrong. Other people come in to get their coats, strewn on my bed, and I start snapping at them, telling them to get the hell out. I start yelling at Christine that I want my room back, I want my life back. As if on cue, Zap proceeds to vomit on a coat that apparently belongs to someone named Roland, which seems like just deserts for coming to my party and being part of my awful night.

I have this palpable, absolute sense that I'm cracking up, that there's really no good reason why, and that—even worse—there's nothing I can do about it. And the thing that's really bugging me, as I lie curled up, is that the scene I'm enacting reminds me of something: It reminds me of my whole life.

Just outside the French doors leading into my room, Christine and Jason and a few other friends—Larissa, Julian, Ron—are conferring. I can hear them, the whispers of discussion, but they don't sound nearly as concerned and conspiratorial as they might have a few years ago. They've seen me this way before, many times. They know I go through this, I survive, I go on, it could be severe premenstrual syndrome, it could be—in this case it probably is—cocaine blues. It could be nothing.

I can imagine Jason saying: Elizabeth's having one of her episodes. I can imagine Christine saying: She's losing it again. I can imagine them all thinking that this is all about a chemical deficiency, that if I'd just take my lithium like a good girl, this wouldn't happen.

By the time I stumble into the bathroom and slam both doors and curl up tight to the floor, I'm certain that there's no way they'll ever understand the philosophical underpinnings of the state I'm in. I know that when I'm on lithium, I'm just fine, that I can cope with the ebb and tide of life, I can handle the setbacks with aplomb, I can be a good sport. But when I'm off the drugs, when my head is clean and clear of this clutter of reason and rationality, what I'm mostly thinking is: Why? Why take it like a man? Why be mature? Why accept adversity? Why surrender with grace the follies of youth? Why put up with the bullshit?

I don't mean to sound like a spoiled brat. I know that into every sunny life a little rain must fall and all that, but in my case the crisis-level hysteria is an all-too-recurring theme. The voices in my head, which I used to think were just passing through, seem to have taken up residence. And I've been on these goddamn pills for years. At first, the idea was to get me going so I could respond to talk therapy, but now it seems clear that my condition is chronic, that I'm going to be on drugs forever if I just want to be barely functional. Prozac alone isn't even enough. I've been off lithium less than a month and I'm already perfectly batty. And I'm starting to wonder if I might not be one of those people like Anne Sexton or Sylvia Plath who are just better off dead, who may live in that bare, minimal sort of way for a certain number of years, may even marry, have kids, create an artistic legacy of sorts, may even be beautiful and enchanting at moments, as both of them supposedly were. But in the end, none of the good was any match for the aching, enduring, suicidal pain. Perhaps I, too, will die young and sad, a corpse with her head in the oven. Scrunched up and crying here on a Saturday night, I can see no other way.

I mean, I don't know if there are any statistics on this, but how long is a person who is on psychotropic drugs supposed to live? How long before your brain, not to mention the rest of you, will begin to mush and deteriorate? I don't think chronically psychotic people tend to make it to the nursing-home-in-Florida phase of life. Or do they? And which is worse: to live that long in this condition or to die young and stay pretty?

I stand up to take out my contact lenses, which are falling out anyway, dripping down a sliding pond of tears. The pair I have on tonight is green, a spare set I got during a buy-one-get-one-free sale, which I wear when I feel like hiding behind a creepy, phony set of eyes. They give me an inanimate appearance like I'm spooked or from another planet or a lifeless Stepford Wife who cooks, cleans, and fucks with a blissful, idiotic smile. Because the lenses are already slipping off of my pupils, it appears that I have two sets of eyes, some sick twist on double vision, and as they slide out I look like a living doll, a horror movie robot whose eyes have fallen out of their sockets.

And then I'm back on the floor.

Jason comes in after everyone has left and urges me to go to bed, says something about how it will all feel better in the morning. And I say, Goddamnit, you asshole! I don't want it to feel better in the morning! I want to deal with the problem and make it better or I want to die right now.

He sits down next to me, but I know he'd rather be with Emily, his girlfriend, or anywhere else. I know he'd rather be washing dishes in the other room or sweeping the floor or gathering cans and bottles for the recycling bin. I know that I'm so awful right now that cleaning is more appealing than sitting with me.

Jason, how long have we known each other? I ask him. What's it been, at least five years, since junior year?

He nods.

And how many times have you seen me like this? How many times have you found me bawling on the floor somewhere? How many times have you found me digging a grapefruit knife into my wrist, screaming that I want to die?

He doesn't answer. He doesn't want to say: Too often.

Jase, it's like twenty-five years already, my whole life. Every so often there's a reprieve, like when Nathan and I first fell in love, or when I first started writing for *The New Yorker*. But then the dullness of everyday kicks in, and I get crazy.

He says something about how when I'm on lithium I seem to be fine. Like that makes it all okay.

I start crying hard, taking little panicked breaths, and when I can talk it's only to say, I don't want to live this life.

I keep crying and Jason just leaves me there.

Julian, who apparently is spending the night because he lost his keys, comes in next. I might as well be Elizabeth Taylor in *Cleopatra,* receiving supplicants on the bathroom floor.

Julian says stuff like, Happiness is a choice, you've got to work toward it. He says it like it's an insight or something.

He says, You've got to believe.

He says, Come on! Cheer up! Pull yourself together!

I can't believe how trite all this is. For a moment I want to step out of myself so I can teach him some better interpersonal skills, so I can help him learn to sound a little more sensitive, more empathic than all this.

But I can't stop crying.

Finally, he picks me up, mumbling something about how all this is nothing a good night's sleep won't cure, saying something about how we're going to go get some lithium in the morning, not understanding that I don't want to feel better in the morning, how that way of life is wearing me out, that what I really want is not to feel this way in the first place.

I keep pushing away from him, demanding that he put me down. I am literally doing what people mean when they say, She went kicking and screaming. Poor Julian. I start poking at his eyes to get him to put me down because that's what I learned to do in a course on self-defense for women. Jason hears me screaming and comes in, and the two of them just kind of force me into bed, and I think that if I don't comply, maybe the men in white coats will come with a straitjacket and take me away, a thought that is momentarily comforting, and ultimately, like everything else, horrifying.

The first time I took an overdose was at summer camp. It must have been 1979, the year I turned twelve, when I had thin thighs, big eyes, peachy breasts, sunburn, and an edge-of-adolescence prettiness that would have made you think nothing could be wrong. Then one day during rest hour, I sat in my bed on the lower bunk, with my friend Lisanne napping just above me, and began to read a book whose epigraph was from Heraclitus: "How can you hide from what never goes away?"

I cannot remember the name of the book, any of its characters or contents, but the quote is indelible, does not come out in the wash, has been on my mind ever since. No matter how many chemicals I have ever used to bleach or sandblast my brain, I know by now, only too well, that you can never get away from yourself because you never go away.

Unless you die. Of course, I wasn't really trying to kill myself that summer. I don't know what I was trying to do. Trying to get my mind off my mind or something. Trying to be not me for a little bit.

So I swallowed about five or ten caplets of Atarax, a prescription allergy medicine I was taking for hay fever. The drug, like most antihistamines, was highly soporific, so I fell asleep for a really long time, long enough to avoid swim in-

struction at the lake and morning prayers by the flagpole
through the end of the week, which was really the point after
all. I couldn't imagine why I was being coerced into all those
activities anyway—the rote motion of newcomb, kickball,
soccer, the breast stroke, making lanyards, all this regimented
activity that seemed meant only to pass a little more time as
we headed, inexorably, toward death. Even then, I was pretty
certain, in my almost-twelve-year-old mind, that life was one
long distraction from the inevitable.

I would watch the other girls in my bunk as they blow-
dried their hair in preparation for night activities, learned to
apply blue eye shadow as they readied themselves to become
teenagers, as they conjured boy problems like, Do you think
he likes me? I watched as they improved their tennis serves
and learned basic lifesaving techniques, as they poured themselves into tight Sasson jeans and covered up with quilted satin
jackets in pink and purple, and I couldn't help wondering
who they were trying to fool. Couldn't they see that all this
was just process—process, process, process—all for naught.

*Everything's plastic, we're all going to die sooner or later, so
what does it matter.* That was my motto.

As it happens, when I took all that Atarax at camp, I fell
so blissfully asleep that no one seemed to notice that anything
was wrong. For once, in fact, nothing *was* wrong. I was, like
the line in a Pink Floyd album I couldn't stop listening to that
year, comfortably numb. I think I must have been sick anyway—nothing more serious than a cold or cough, and had
been staying in bed a lot. I didn't really want to go back to
the infirmary, where gooey grape-flavored Dimetapp was
universally recognized to be the cure for all ills. Perhaps it
seemed to everyone that I was recovering from a summer flu
or something like that. Or maybe they took my bed-bound
state for granted, just as my classmates at school no longer
expected me to be at lunch, had come to accept that I would

be hiding in the locker room carving razor cuts onto my legs, playing with my own blood, as if that's what everyone else was doing between 12:15 and 1:00 P.M. Every time one of the counselors tried to prod me out of bed, I was too passed out, and they probably thought it was easier just to leave me alone. It's not like I was anyone's pet.

Eventually, I think maybe Lisanne got to worrying. The lump of my body under woolen blankets had become a strange fixture in the room. After a few days, the head counselor came to see me in my little cot, I think to encourage me to see a doctor. I thought to tell her that I would love nothing more than to receive medical attention—*any* attention would be just fine with me—but I was too incapacitated to move.

"So how are you feeling today?" she asked as she sat down at my feet, sliding a clipboard with schedules of activities on it beside her. Through a blur in my eyes, I looked down at her legs, full of varicose veins. She was wearing Keds that were perfectly white, as if they'd never been worn before.

"I'm fine."

"Do you think you'll want to go play volleyball with your bunk this morning?"

"No." Did I *look* like I wanted to play volleyball, lying here and shivering under a thick wool army blanket in the middle of July?

"Well then," she continued, like it was normal, "you should probably see the nurse so we can figure out what's wrong with you. Are you feverish?" She pressed her hand to my forehead, which my mother once told me was not a reliable predictor of anything, just a gesture of maternal authority. "No, no." She shook her head. "If anything, you feel cold. That's probably because you haven't been eating."

I wondered how much she knew about me, if she'd been privy to my files, or if they even kept such things at summer camp. Did she know that I really wasn't supposed to be here at all? Did she understand that it was just that my mother sent me here for an eight-week reprieve from single parenthood? Did she know that we had no money, that I was here as some sort of charity case, that they'd taken me because my mother worked too hard for too little and didn't know what else to do with me when school was out? Did she understand that this was all a big mistake?

"Look, I'm really not sick," I leveled with her. I was hoping that if I told her the truth about what was wrong with me she'd insist that my mother come get me this minute, which was all I really wanted. "I just have allergies, really bad allergies, and the other day I took some of my medication, and I must have taken too much because I haven't been able to move ever since."

"What kind was it?"

I reached into the cubby beside my bed where I kept tapes and books and pills, and flashed the near-empty bottle in front of her, shaking it like a baby's rattle. "Atarax. My doctor gave it to me."

"I see." Since I wasn't even twelve yet, she couldn't blame this on adolescent angst. She really couldn't blame this on much of anything. Neither could I.

I found myself wanting to explain it to her, to this middle-aged woman with the kind of haircut you call a hairdo, which needed to be set in rollers every night, who had a name like Agnes or Harriet, a name that even predated my mother's generation. I wanted to open up the vial and show her the Atarax, let her see that the white childproof cap could not fool this child. I wanted to show her the solid black pills and how pretty they were. They looked like what I imagined black beauties must look like. They were so tempting, their appearance was so subversive, that it was almost impossible for me to take just one. These little black death angels

were *meant* to kill you. Never mind that they were just antihistamines, perhaps no stronger than what you get over the
counter. Never mind that the person who prescribed them
was thinking only of the pollen that was swelling my eyes and
stuffing up my nasal passages. Never mind.

There was no way I could have explained my chronic
moroseness to the head counselor, no way I could tell her
how I had already alienated most of my bunkmates—who
were themselves into Donna Summer and Sister Sledge and
arguing over who got to be John Travolta and who got to be
Olivia Newton-John in their lip-sync renditions of *Grease*—
by playing the Velvet Underground on my crappy little tape
recorder late into the night. How could they possibly understand why it made no sense to me to listen to disco music and
dance around the cabin when I could lie on the concrete floor
with just the single bulb of bathroom light while Lou Reed's
voice would lure me into a life of nihilism?

There was no way the head counselor or anyone else
would ever understand that I didn't like being this way. How
jealous I was of all the other girls who were boy crazy and
loud and fun. How much I wanted to flip my hair and flirt
and be rowdy but somehow just *couldn't*—didn't dare—even
try anymore. How awful it would be for me when it was time
to celebrate my birthday in a couple of weeks with a frosted
cake at dinnertime. How horrible it would be when everyone
sang and I blew out the candles, all the while everyone knowing that this was an elaborate act of pity or propriety, that it
had nothing to do with anyone really being my friend. There
was no way I could ever get them or the head counselor or
anyone here who didn't know me from before to believe that
it wasn't always like this, that I had convinced all the girls in
my first-grade class that I was their boss (it was a simple swin-
dle, a basic Ponzi scheme: if they didn't agree to accept me
as their boss, none of the people I'd already taken in would

be allowed to be their friends), that the teacher had to meet with the class as a group to explain that we were all free, that there was no such thing as a boss, and still my friends would not renounce me as their leader. How could I ever get her to see that I'd been the class bully, I'd been popular, I'd been in Pampers commercials at six months, had done Hi-C and Starburst ads later, had written a series of pet care books at age six, had adapted "Murders in the Rue Morgue" into a play at age seven, had turned construction paper and Magic Markers and tempera paint into an illustrated chapbook called *Penny the Penguin* at age eight, that no one in her right mind would ever have believed I'd come to this: eleven and almost gone.

My mother had attributed the changes in me to menarche, as if menstrual blood made everyone crazy, as if this were just a phase and I could still go to summer camp like I was okay after all. If my mom couldn't see what was happening, there was no way I could confide in this antediluvian head counselor, who seemed to have reached the safe verdict that I had mistakenly taken more pills than I should have, that perhaps the incessant rain was giving me such bad hay fever I'd gone a little overboard. "You realize you're supposed to give any prescription drugs to the nurse," she said, as if it mattered anymore. "You were supposed to do that at the beginning of the summer. She would have been able to administer these correctly."

I should have said, *Do I look like I give a shit about having my pills ad-fucking-ministered correctly? Do I?*

My little chat with the head counselor never really amounted to much. I saw her speak in hushed tones to my immediate counselors about why I was sleeping so much, and the next day one of the more senior medical people came to see me, but life went on as usual.

My parents never came charging up to the Pocono

Mountains to bring me back home. In fact, the way the head counselor looked at the Atarax bottle, you'd have thought that the pills were a danger to me and not, as was the case, that I was dangerous to myself. Once I got back home, my mother never mentioned the Atarax incident to me. My father, in one of our Saturday afternoon visits, which were dwindling to no more than one or two a month, did manage to express some concern. But I think everyone thought it was just a mistake, a little kid plays with matches and gets burned, a preteen has slightly more complex tools to mess with, takes too many pills, dozes (doses?) off for a little too long. It happens.

Monday morning, two days after the party, I am back at the Fifth Avenue Crack House, a.k.a. Dr. Ira's office. It's actually about three in the afternoon, but that's early for me.

Dr. Ira is berating me for going off lithium without discussing it with him first. I explain that I panicked, the Graves' disease and all. He explains that the blood tests I get every couple of months monitor me so closely that we would know if there were a problem long before it got out of hand, that we could take necessary steps in advance of such an emergency. He's making sense. I can't and don't argue. Besides, he tells me that the results on a second set of blood levels came out perfectly normal. He thinks the mistake was all about a misplaced decimal point, a computer error that turned 1.4 into 14. Right now, the TSH level is a perfectly average 1.38.

Of course, I don't know what any of these numbers mean, don't really want to ask. But I can't pull myself away from a nagging suspicion that it just can't be this simple. What I mean is this: Prozac has rather minimal side effects, the lithium has a few more, but basically the pair keep me functioning as a sane human being, at least most of the time. And I can't help feeling that anything that works so effectively, that's so transformative, has got to be hurting me at another end, maybe sometime further down the road.

I can just hear the words *inoperable brain cancer* being whispered to me by some physician twenty years from now.

I mean, the law of conservation says that no matter or energy is ever destroyed, it's only converted into something else, and I still can't say exactly how my depression has metamorphosed. My guess is it's still hanging out in my head, doing deadly things to my gray matter, or worse, that it's just waiting for the clock on this Prozac stuff to run out so that it can attack again, send me back into a state of catatonia, just like those characters in the movie *Awakenings* who fall back into their pre-L-dopa stupor after just a few months.

Every time I come in for an appointment, I run my misgivings by Dr. Ira. I say something like: Come on, level with me, anything that works this well has got to have some unknown downside.

Or, taking another tack: Look, let's face it, I was one of the first people to be put on Prozac after the FDA approved it. Who's to say that I won't be the test case that proves it causes, well, um, say—*inoperable brain cancer?*

He says a bunch of reassuring things, explains over and over again how carefully he is monitoring me—all the while admitting that psychopharmacology is more art than science, that he and his colleagues are all basically shooting in the dark. And he acts as if a million doctors didn't say the same things to women about DES, about the IUD, about silicone breast implants, as if they didn't once claim that Valium was a non-addictive tranquilizer and that Halcion was a miracle sleeping pill. As if class-action suits against pharmaceutical companies were not fairly routine by now.

Just the same, I am leaving for Miami Beach the next day, am sufficiently sick of being miserable that I take two little green and white Prozac capsules when I leave his office, and dutifully resume taking a twice-daily dose of lithium, also downing twenty milligrams of Inderal each day—a beta-blocker normally used to lower blood pressure—because I need it to counteract the hand shaking and the other tremorous side effects of lithium. Taking drugs breeds taking more drugs.

And I can't believe, looking at myself in the mirror, seeing what to all eyes must appear to be a young and healthy twenty-five-year-old with flushed skin and visible biceps—I can't believe anyone in his right mind would deny that these are just too damn many pills.

1

Full of Promise

✳ ✳ ✳

And suddenly, as he noted the fine shades of manner
by which she harmonized herself with her surroundings, it flashed on him that, to need such adroit han-
dling, the situation must indeed be desperate.

EDITH WHARTON
The House of Mirth

Some catastrophic situations invite clarity, explode in split
moments: You smash your hand through a windowpane and
then there is blood and shattered glass stained with red all
over the place; you fall out a window and break some bones
and scrape some skin. Stitches and casts and bandages and
antiseptic solve and salve the wounds. But depression is not
a sudden disaster. It is more like a cancer: At first its tumorous
mass is not even noticeable to the careful eye, and then one
day—wham!—there is a huge, deadly seven-pound lump
lodged in your brain or your stomach or your shoulder blade,
and this thing that your own body has produced is actually
trying to kill you. Depression is a lot like that: Slowly, over
the years, the data will accumulate in your heart and mind, a
computer program for total negativity will build into your
system, making life feel more and more unbearable. But you
won't even notice it coming on, thinking that it is somehow
normal, something about getting older, about turning eight

or turning twelve or turning fifteen, and then one day you realize that your entire life is just awful, not worth living, a horror and a black blot on the white terrain of human existence. One morning you wake up afraid you are going to live.

In my case, I was not frightened in the least bit at the thought that I might live because I was certain, quite certain, that I was already dead. The actual dying part, the withering away of my physical body, was a mere formality. My spirit, my emotional being, whatever you want to call all that inner turmoil that has nothing to do with physical existence, were long gone, dead and gone, and only a mass of the most fucking god-awful excruciating pain like a pair of boiling hot tongs clamped tight around my spine and pressing on all my nerves was left in its wake.

That's the thing I want to make clear about depression: It's got nothing at all to do with life. In the course of life, there is sadness and pain and sorrow, all of which, in their right time and season, are normal—unpleasant, but normal. Depression is in an altogether different zone because it involves a complete absence: absence of affect, absence of feeling, absence of response, absence of interest. The pain you feel in the course of a major clinical depression is an attempt on nature's part (nature, after all, abhors a vacuum) to fill up the empty space. But for all intents and purposes, the deeply depressed are just the walking, waking dead.

And the scariest part is that if you ask anyone in the throes of depression how he got there, to pin down the turning point, he'll never know. There is a classic moment in *The Sun Also Rises* when someone asks Mike Campbell how he went bankrupt, and all he can say in response is, "Gradually and then suddenly." When someone asks how I lost my mind, that is all I can say too.

★   ★   ★

It seems to me that I was about eleven when it happened. Maybe I was ten or maybe I was twelve, but it was somewhere in my preadolescence. In other words, since puberty hadn't kicked in yet, no one was expecting it.

I remember the exact date, December 5, 1978, when I was eleven, and noticed some dry brown spots that were obviously blood on my little white cotton briefs. I met my mother at Bloomingdale's that night—Bloomingdale's to look, Alexander's to buy was our rule—in search of a winter coat, and I told her about the stains in my panties, told her I thought maybe I had my period (I knew about menstruation from reading *Lifecycle* books with Lisanne in elementary school, which at the time I was still in), and all she could say was, Oh no. Maybe afterward she said something like, God help me, the trouble has just begun. But whatever she said gave me the strong and distinct impression that suddenly I was going to become difficult and morose, which already seemed to be happening.

When I try to understand where I made a bad turn, how I stupidly meandered down the wrong road in the fork of life, I can't shake the sense that being born smack in the middle of the Summer of Love (July 31, 1967), with the confluence of social revolutions from no-fault divorce to feminism to free love to Vietnam—and their eventual displacement by punk rock and Reaganomics—all had something to do with it. I hate to think that personal development, with its template of idiosyncrasies, can be reduced to explanations as simple as "it was the times," but the sixties counterculture—along with its alter ego, eighties greed—has imprinted itself all over me.

Even so, I wasn't raised by some wasted, crazed hippie parents who smoked pot in Central Park while carrying me in a tie-dyed Snugli, took me to Woodstock at age two, and by virtue of their reckless postadolescent irresponsibility, managed to screw me up but good. Nothing could be further from the truth. My mom was a die-hard Republican who voted for Nixon three times, who wanted them to escalate the Vietnam War effort, and who went to see William F. Buckley speak while she was an undergraduate at Cornell in the early sixties. As she tells it, so few students at the liberal college she attended showed up at the lecture that she threw her coat across several seats to make it look as if more were coming. (My mom, by the way, is the only person I know at this point who thinks Oliver North is a hero.) My dad was apolitical, had absolutely no professional aspirations, and worked as a low-level employee at a large corporation. He had short hair and wore Buddy Holly nerd glasses, read Isaac Asimov, and listened to Tony Bennett. The closest thing we ever had to a political discussion was sometime when I was about eight and he told me it was crappy of President Ford to pardon Nixon because lying was really bad. Basically, my parents had no unconventional tendencies, though they occasionally bought bad Mary Travers albums.

My parents, like the progenitors of most people my age, were not those freewheeling, footloose and fancy-free baby boomers who made the sixties happen. They were just an itty bit too old for that, born in 1939 and 1940 instead of 1944 and 1945 (in an accelerated culture, five years makes a world of difference). For the most part, the parents of my contemporaries were done with college and had moved onto the workaday world by the early sixties, several years before the campus uprisings, the antiwar activities, and the emerging sex-drugs-rock-and-roll culture had become a pervasive force.

By the time the radical sixties hit their home bases, we, the kids, were already born, and our parents found themselves stuck between an entrenched belief that children needed to be raised in a traditional household, and a new sense that anything was possible, that the alternative lifestyle was out there for the asking. There they were, in marriages they once thought were a necessity and with children they'd had almost by accident in a world that was suddenly saying, *No necessities! No accidents! Drop everything!* A little too old to take full advantage of the cultural revolution, our parents just got all the fallout. Freedom hit them obliquely, and invidiously, rather than head-on. Instead of waiting longer to get married, our parents got divorced; instead of becoming feminists, our mothers were left to become displaced homemakers. A lot of unhappy situations were dissolved by people who were not quite young or free (read: childless) enough to start again. And their discontent, their stuck-ness, was played out on their children. Sharing kids with a person you have come to despise must be a bit like getting caught in a messy car wreck and then being forced to spend the rest of your life paying visits to the paraplegic in the other vehicle: You are never allowed to forget your mistake.

My parents are a perfect case in point. Lord knows whatever possessed them to get married in the first place. It probably had something to do with the fact that my mom was raised with many of her first cousins, and all of them were getting married, so it seemed like the thing to do. And from her point of view, back in the early sixties, marriage was the only way she could get out of her parents' house. She'd gone to Cornell to be an architect, but her mother told her that all she could be was an architect's *secretary*, so she majored in art history with that goal in mind. She'd spent a junior year abroad at the Sorbonne and did all the studiedly adventurous things a nice Jewish girl from Long Island can do in Paris— rented a motorbike, wore a black cape, dated some nobleman type—but once she got out of college, she moved back home and was expected to stay there until she moved into her husband's house. (Certainly there were many bolder women who defied this expectation, who took efficiencies and railroad flats with girlfriends in the city, who worked and dated and went to theater openings and lectures—but my mom was not one of them.) She took a job in the executive training program at Macy's, and one day while she was riding the escalator up from the main floor to the mezzanine, she passed my father, who was riding down. They were wed less than a year later.

My parents did weird things after they got married. My dad got a job at IBM and they moved to Poughkeepsie, where my mom went nuts with boredom and bought herself a pet monkey named Percy. Eventually she got pregnant with me, decided a baby was better than a monkey, and moved down to New York City because she could not bear another day in a town that was half Vassar College, half IBM. My father followed, I was born, they fought, they were miserable, he refused to get a college degree, they fought some more, and then one day I wouldn't stop crying. My mom called my dad at work to say that if he didn't come home immediately and figure out how to get me to calm down, she was going to defenestrate me. Whatever my father did when he got to the apartment must have worked, because I'm still alive today, but I think that moment marked the end of their marriage. Sometime after that, my parents were trying to hang a picture in the apartment, and my mom absolutely refused to hold the nail in place while he hammered it into the wall; she was sure he was going to misfire and bang her fingers, and she would end up bruised and broken. After that, they went to a marriage counselor they read about in *Time* magazine who made them play with toy trains to see how their relationship worked. Something about the way they put things together on the tracks made him conclude it was hopeless. My mom threw my dad out of the house, and he went home to his mother and his diabetic, alcoholic father in their cinder-block apartment complex in Brighton Beach, and that was the end.

This marriage could have peacefully ceased to be one fine day with an understanding that it was just a mistake, they were just two foolish kids playing house. Problem was, they had a child, and for many years after they split up, I became the battlefield on which all their ideological differences were fought. This was New York City in the late sixties: Harlem had burned down, Columbia University was shut down, Central Park had become an international center of love-ins and be-ins and drug-ins, and my mom was petrified about being a single mother with a deadbeat ex-husband. She sent me to the synagogue nursery school, thinking this would provide me with some sense of community and stability, while my dad, who turned up to see me about once a week, would talk to me about atheism, insisting I eat lobster and ham and other nonkosher foods that I was taught were not allowed. A daily Valium doser, my dad would spend most of our Saturday afternoon visits sleeping, leaving me to watch TV or paint with watercolors or call my mom to say, *Daddy won't move, I think he's dead.* (One time we went to see *The Last Waltz*, and he passed out. I couldn't get him to budge, so we sat through the movie three times; I think this might explain my abiding crush on Robbie Robertson.)

For years, my mom tugged toward trying to give me a solid, middle-class, traditional upbringing, while my father would tell me that I should just be an artist or a poet or live off the land, or some such thing. But as arty and expansive as his ideas may have sounded, my father's attitude and lassitude were not grounded in any sort of sixties collegiate bohemian philosophy of live and let live: He came from a background that was more blue collar-immigrant than anything else. And instead of college, he'd done time in the U.S. Army. He was not cool or groovy at all, just a fuckup. So while my mom, struggling with her part-time income and trying to take care of me, was frantic to keep at least a toehold in the bourgeoisie, my dad was working overtime (or actually, not *gainfully* working much at all) to stay the hell out of it. This went on, back and forth, for years, until it was clear that all three of us were caught mostly in the confusing crossfire of changing times, and what little foundation my parents could possibly give me was shattered and scattered by conflict.

I don't doubt that there might have been another kind of awfulness in being born to a couple of hippie druggies or politicos (I'm sure the kids a few years my junior have their own lists of gripes), but I'm convinced that it was worse to have grown up in revolutionary times, in the midst of a wildly vibrant city like New York, raised by people who were not really involved or engaged in the culture. Does anyone really want to be a wallflower at the orgy? My mom was desperate to shelter me from what she perceived as sheer lunacy, and my dad, who began loading up on tranquilizers shortly after the divorce, was just plain indifferent. I really believe that had either of them had any strong convictions or values to pass on to me, my worldview might have emerged as more sanguine than sanguinary. Instead, all they had to offer me was their fear: My mom feared the outside world and my dad feared me and my mom; we lived in a paranoid household in which everyone defined his own enemies and pretty soon everyone was implicated.

One day, when I was about ten, my father told me that he had never wanted to have a kid with my mom, that their marriage was for shit and he had thought a child was a bad idea. But once she got pregnant, he added, he was most de-lighted. He said that my mother wanted to have an abortion, that she'd gotten as far as the gynecologist's office and was all set to have a D and C, and that he physically restrained her to prevent the process. Later, when I told my mother about this conversation, she began to cry and said that the opposite was true: She wanted me and *he* didn't. Given that she was the custodial parent, took care of me and loved me while he slept through most of my childhood and ran away without leaving a trace when I was fourteen, I must assume she is telling the truth. But who really cares? Some people are born to single mothers and turn out just fine. I don't think it matters how many parents you've got, so long as the ones who are around make their presence felt in a positive way. But I got two parents who were constantly at odds with each other, and all they gave me was an empty foundation that split down the middle of my empty, anguished self.

They were separated and divorced before I was two.

My only memory of my father living in the same place as me: I am, of course, just a toddler. I wander into my parents' bedroom and find my father still lying there in the queen-size bed under the covers, his glasses perched on his nose kind of crookedly, his head bent to one side, kind of askew. He looks over at me but not really. Or maybe not at all. I have a pacifier plugged in my mouth, one of about thirty that I keep and name, one of about thirty that I stay up all night playing with, as I lie in the folds of covers forming a castle with my knees bent. My dad is still half asleep, forcing himself to stay awake because Mommy is already up and about, already making omelettes and café au lait. The sheets on the bed are pink with maroon and white diagonal stripes of varying thicknesses, definitely the fashion, meant to look a bit like a Frank Stella painting or a Vidal Sassoon geometric cut. They are so straight and solid, and my dad is so twisted and gelatinous.

On the wall is a poster, popular in the late sixties, of a broken heart held together by a Band-Aid, as if things could be fixed this easily (or perhaps it is making fun of that notion). At any rate, my father, still beardless at this point, is pushing himself up with his hands to sit against the black antique wrought-iron headboard.

This is my only memory of Daddy at home. In all my early memories of him, he is sleeping or just waking up or about to go to sleep. Frequently, during our Saturday visits after the split, my father would take me for Chinese food, and afterward we would retreat to his studio walk-up, turn on the TV, and I would watch while he fell asleep. Usually on weekend afternoons, all that was on were college sports—I recall many NCAA championships—which didn't interest me, and Star Trek reruns, which confused me (my dad, on the other hand, is a hopeless Trekkie, but he slept through all of this anyway). Occasionally there'd be a movie about the Donner Party or some other gruesome historical event. Sometimes he'd get me a model airplane or car to construct and paint with bullet gray enamel and the war stripes of the Allies or the Axis countries. I am the only girl I know who builds model vehicles, and it is only because it is all he gives me to do while he sleeps. Sometimes I tap him and try to get him to help me fit a wing in place or paint a tight crevice in a silver fender, but he doesn't budge.

I don't take it personally that my father snoozes through our visits. After all, how much can you really say to a little kid, and probably we'd already covered it at lunch. Later on, when I am old enough to know about these things, I tell my mom that I think he's narcoleptic, and she says that all men are like that, that the army teaches men to be able to sleep anywhere so they do. When I am old enough to ask my father about it, when I wonder why he sleeps through our little bit of quality time together, he just speaks of nerves—of nerves and Valium. Librium and Miltown and whatever else too.

When I am three, my mother goes to Israel for three weeks, ostensibly to look into living there. Though we aren't particularly religious, she thinks that maybe the Middle East, where the war zones are mostly outside the home, is a more stable place to raise a child. My father tells me that she has gone away because she is losing her mind, but whatever the reason, Daddy comes to stay with me for the time being. I think this setup is great because it means I never have to get to nursery school on time: My father sleeps right through the morning.

He sleeps on the green sofa bed in the living room (apparently it is too unpleasant to stay in the bed he once shared with Mommy), and every morning I rise at the crack of dawn and play with my coloring books or read Dr. Seuss or ride on my rocking horse and watch Captain Kangaroo and wait for him to get up and make me breakfast. Hours go by. Eventually it seems like lunchtime and I am so hungry that I tiptoe into the living room, stand there staring at him, hoping the power of my gaze will wake him. It doesn't.

Finally, I approach the bed, over at the part where his face rests and the springs and coils connect the mattress to the couch, and I take my little fingers and carefully peel his eye open as if I were a police officer examining a corpse at the scene of the crime. At first, I expose just the white, but eventually the iris and pupil roll into view, and I in turn roll into his view, and he looks a little stunned, like this is not quite what he expected, like who is this stranger standing over his face, or like maybe he's been driving for a long time and he somehow has picked up the wrong hitchhiker.

And I say, Daddy, it's me.

For three weeks straight, I arrive at school at least three hours late, and every time it happens, Patti, the teacher, just laughs. My dad does his imitation of Donald Duck for me and the other kids, and then he is gone.

The first time I see any therapist—and there have been so many first times—there are certain routine questions we must go through. There is the usual medical trivia: Are you allergic to penicillin? Whom do we contact in an emergency? Are you on any drugs? And then there's all the family stuff: not the anecdotal kind that is the bulk of therapy itself, but things like, Is there any history of depression in your family? At first, I always forget about everyone else, about my cousins who tried to kill themselves and about my great grandmother who died in an asylum and about my grandfather the alcoholic and about my grandmother with the terrible melancholia and about my father who was obviously very fucked up—I always forget about all these people and say, *I'm the only one*. It's not an act. I just honestly don't think of any of these people as really related to me because they're all on my dad's side, and I hardly feel like he's in my family.

Pamela, my first cousin, tried to end it all by slitting her wrists, or at least so the story goes. I remember hearing about all the blood and mess, but it was years later when my dad mentioned the suicide attempt to me, adding that her brother had also tried, but with drugs I think, and by then the indelible impression I had always had of my cousins as rather ordinary bland blond kids was too well developed for the information to register. Besides, almost nothing my father told me ever really stuck because I was convinced that he was nuts himself.

I could just as easily dismiss the thing about my great grandmother dying in the asylum as insignificant. After all, back then they put women away for wanting to work for a living or for asking for a divorce. Or she could have had tuberculosis or typhoid, besides. And it was hard to know that there was anything particularly wrong with my grandfather beyond being old and sickly because that's all he was by the time I came along. It wasn't until he died and we didn't go to the funeral that my dad told me what a mean drunk he was, that he beat my grandmother, and that one night my dad broke his father's ribs trying to kill him (who knows if any of this is true). To me, Grandpa Saul was just a docile old man. And Grandma Dorothy, well, she surely must have had an awful life, but I knew her only as the old lady who made chicken soup for me on the rare occasions my father took me to visit (he, of course, would spend the time asleep in a lounge chair in front of the television set) her little apartment full of fake wood furniture, pile carpet, impressionistic wallpaper, with a view of the Cyclone roller coaster in Coney Island.

My grandmother always seemed like any other oversolicitous, doting Jewish mother to me.

And my dad—I just thought he was really tired.

It never occurred to me that any of this was a problem.

But now, years later, I must admit that unhappiness seems to run in the family, there have been so many generations of it on my dad's side that I wonder why someone doesn't just—I don't know how—put a stop to it. I don't know why someone doesn't throw a big black umbrella over our heads and pull us all in out of the rain.

So I mention the family history of depression to every new therapist when it finally occurs to me, and they always feel obligated to point out the genetic component of mental illness. But then I'll tell them a little bit about my immediate family background, and sooner or later, as the narrative continues, they're sure to say something like, *No wonder you're so depressed*, like it's the most obvious response. They react as if my family situation was particularly alarming and troublesome, as opposed to what it actually is in this day and age: perfectly normal. I mean, I think about my development and I feel like a Census Bureau statistic or some sort of case study on the changing nature of the American family in the late twentieth century. My parents are divorced, I grew up in a female-headed household, my mother was always unemployed or marginally employed, my father was always uninvolved or marginally involved in my life. There was never enough money for anything, my mom had to sue my dad for unpaid child support and unpaid medical bills, my dad eventually disappeared. But all this information is no more outstanding than the plot of an Ann Beattie novel. Or maybe it's not even that interesting.

In college, I can remember sitting around dorm rooms and coffeehouses late at night during my freshman year comparing family horror stories with my new friends. We'd almost be competitive about whose father was the least responsible (Jordana would always complain that her dad had enough money for fine wines and a Park Avenue apartment, but he still never so much as took her to dinner), or whose mother was the most scattered, hysterical, or just plain out of it from being overburdened with parenting duties (I always won that contest). It was always interesting to see who could hold the record for not communicating with the noncustodial parent (almost always the father) the longest, either because he'd gotten remarried and moved to San Diego or because he was just a cut-rate shithead who'd skipped town for no particular reason.

The more children of divorce I have met over the years, the more common and trivial my own family history starts to seem. And I always feel so stupid sitting in therapy talking about my problems because, Jesus Christ, so what? I can't equate the amount of pain and misery and despair I have suffered and endured as a depressive with the events of my life, which just seem so common. My reaction has been uncommonly strong, but really, it seems wrong to blame a statistical fact of life for any of it.

When you consider the widespread nature of depression—particularly among people my age—it all becomes completely numbing, like so much pounding on a frozen, paralyzed limb that bruises but no longer feels. The particulars of what has driven this or that person to Zoloft, Paxil, or Prozac, or the reasons that some other person believes herself to be suffering from a major depression, seem less significant than the simple fact of it. To ask anyone how he happened to fall into a state of despair always involves new variations on the same myriad mix of family history. There is always divorce, death, drunkenness, drug abuse and whatnot in any of several permutations. I mean, is there anybody out there who *doesn't* think her family is dysfunctional?

★ ★ ★

But surely my dad couldn't have always slept through our visits. After all, he was an avid photographer, he loved his Nikon, and I was his favorite subject. The only sure way to keep him awake was to hand him a camera. His preschool pictures of me are the best: as a two-year-old chasing a squirrel in Central Park; drinking from a water fountain in the zoo; sitting on the desk at my mother's office, my dress inadvertently hiked up so much that my underwear shows; wearing my mom's shoes and sunglasses around the house; walking the dog. There is even one particular shot of me sitting cross-legged on a park bench in stretchy shorts and a white T-shirt with pigtails and thick bangs and Indian beads around my neck, and a cryptic, pensive expression on my face. One of my cheeks is puffed out, like I'm bored or confused. People thought that picture was so cute that it ended up on a greeting card with typed haiku-ish words on it saying, "People like me like people like you." Apparently it sold well in California.

One day while he was taking pictures of me in the Central Park zoo (I must have been only two or three), I asked my dad when he was coming back home.

"Honey, I'm not," he said. I guess I was looking down at the ground at this point because I remember how the zoo was paved with gray hexagonal bricks.

"But Mommy says you are," I protested.

"I'm sure Mommy didn't say that." He paused, looked exhausted, like he was going to pass out. "Mommy and I are going to live apart from now on, which we tried to explain to you." As an afterthought, he added, "Which doesn't mean I love you any less."

"But, Daddy," I persisted, "Mommy told me to tell you that if you want to come back home, she wants you to come back."

"I'm sure that's not true."

And, of course, it wasn't.

During that same period—early in their separation, when they were still making valiant efforts at civility—my father would some-

times babysit for me on nights when my mom went out. Sometimes he'd bring along his girlfriend, soon to be my stepmother, Elinor, and I would play with the huge, brightly colored Pucci scarves that she wore with her turtlenecks, blindfolding myself or fondling the soft silk. Our apartment had a long, narrow, closet-lined hallway, and one of my favorite activities was to stand on my father's feet as he held my arms above my head for balance, and walk on his shoes with him through the hall, quite literally walking in his footsteps. And when it was time for me to go to sleep, I would make my father leave those same shoes, rusty brown half boots, in the hallway outside my bedroom door. I wanted them to be there so I could look out and know he was still there. It was like I knew he was planning to disappear on me sometime.

Before I went to bed, I always used to ask my dad and Elinor when they were going to get married. Sometimes I'd tell them I was going to fire them both if they didn't do it soon. Not having any idea really what a normal family was like, I thought it was pretty neat that my dad was going to be married and I would get to go to a real wedding—as opposed to the one I'd performed for my Barbie and Ken dolls, or the ceremony I'd had with Mark Cooper in nursery school when he said that I could be Catwoman if he could be Batman, which basically meant that I wouldn't tell on him when he tried to beat me up during rest hour. After all these mock weddings, I think I was hoping to be a flower girl and get a new dress. I guess it never occurred to me that he and Elinor would ever omit me from the wedding altogether: the ceremony, the reception, the dinner afterward. Mommy said that Daddy must have thought that was the best thing to do. But I was only five years old, and all I knew was that there was a party I hadn't been asked to.

I think it was about the time of my dad's second marriage that I first began to have a sense of people disappearing.

My mother and I moved to the Upper West Side, and I became part of a whole new breed—or, at any rate, a whole new brand—of child that seemed to have emerged from the collective gene pool at about that time. While that section of Manhattan has since become a haven for yuppies and recent college graduates, when I was little it was full of single mothers, religious Jews, ballerinas, intellectual types that you'd see in Woody Allen movies, and the occasional *artiste*. The playground in Central Park was full of hippie housewives dressed in clogs and blue jeans, sitting and watching their children, who, as a rule, were wise beyond their years, sophisticated waifs in love beads and Danskin pants, patchwork versions of hip who were mouthy and clever, who didn't actually know what sex was or where babies came from but still used words like *sexy* or *fuck you* with the knowing, mimicking voices of children who have spent far too much time in the company of adults.

I think the type is epitomized by the daughter in the film *The Goodbye Girl*. She is far more levelheaded and reasonable than her dancer-mom, who is juggling romance and rent and a career and an aching back with a certain unflappable humor that always seems on the verge of giving way to a complete emotional breakdown. Marsha Mason is meant to come across as, without a doubt, a good and responsible mother—in fact she is clearly nuts about her daughter and has absolutely no negligent or abusive tendencies—but she is, basically, in over her head. That was what my mom was like: Somehow, the bills always got paid, the babysitter always got paid, the private school scholarships always came through, and she always found the odd bit of part-time work that kept us fed and clothed. But it was so very precarious. I always had the vague sense that we were one paycheck or one man or one job away from welfare. I can remember standing on line with my mom to collect unemployment benefits, and I can remember listening to her plead with my father to send me to a *real* doctor, that there was no way she was going to take me to some clinic even if he thought it was good enough. Money, or the lack of it, pervaded the house as only something that is absent can.

But in the midst of this strange and insecure household, my mom and I, much like the mother and daughter in *The Goodbye Girl*, managed to have tons of fun, to be better as pals than we ever were as parent and child. Since I went to a Jewish school where the divorce rate among parents was fairly low (that was the main reason my mom sent me there), I would visit friends' homes and find myself amazed at how glum things seemed compared to life at our apartment. The fathers always seemed so old and distant and unapproachable, wearing their business suits and showing up in the kids' bedrooms only to offer discipline or help with homework. They were already graying and paunchy, and they usually smelled bad, in that certain fatherly way; the moms quite simply lacked style, were dowdy and schoolmarmish, and they often smelled bad to me as well. They were no fun, and they never seemed like the kind of people you could call by their first names no matter how old you were. The sheer joy of having kids seemed completely lost on them. They did not *get down* with parenthood. My mom, on the other hand, really hung out with me whenever she was at home, helping me fill in the patterns on the Lite-Brite or dunking Oreo cookies in milk with me or dancing around the living room with me while we played *Free to Be You and Me*.

Alone with babysitters a fair amount of time, I would often befriend the teenage girls who came around to watch me while my mom worked. They all seemed to enjoy braiding my long, long hair or teaching me how to draw with charcoal and pastels, and not just Magic Markers. I'd ask about their boyfriends and try to convince them to invite them over for me to check out. One of my babysitters had a father who was a drunk and held us locked in the apartment in a state of holy terror for several hours as he banged on the door and threatened to kill us both. Another babysitter had an older brother who was studying to be a priest. Years later I found out that she'd become a crack addict and had had two babies out of wedlock.

But it didn't much matter who was given the task of watching me for the few hours between the end of the school day and my mother's return from work because I was always perfectly content to be left alone with one of my many odd projects, whether it was breeding grasshoppers that I'd brought home with me from day camp, or writing an illustrated series of books about different kinds of animals, or just sitting around with my math workbooks and zooming ahead through multiplication and division when everyone else in first grade was still learning how to add and subtract. My inner resources were so thorough and complete that I often had no idea what to do with other children. They all seemed so juvenile to me, especially compared to my mom or to my babysitters like Nelsa and Kristina and Cynthia, who were already in high school and wore bell-bottom jeans with painted-on flower appliqués on the pockets and thighs.

You see, until the very moment when I first broke down at age eleven, I was a golden girl in spite of everything. True, my parents were a little out of it and at each other's throats all the time, but I had more than compensated for that by being adorable and charming in the way of precocious little girls, by doing so well in school, by being stubborn and domineering, by being so fucking persistent.

While we didn't keep a kosher home, I somehow managed to win the school Brochos Bee, the Jewish equivalent of a spelling bee, five years in a row. Instead of spelling words, I had to know what blessings to say on different foods. I retired from this rather odd competition after winning the national contest, against boys with earlocks and girls who wore long sleeves and thick tights in June. For my Bible courses, I would rack up extra-credit points by learning various Hebrew passages by heart and reciting them in class. It always amazed teachers that no one at home could speak or read Hebrew, that I seemed to be tutoring myself (eventually, my mom felt left out and took lessons); the educators seemed unable to comprehend the overwhelming sense of invincibleness I possessed. No one could ever have imagined that as a child I was completely convinced that I could do anything on earth I wanted to. By the time I was in seventh grade, they set up a separate class for me, my friend Dinah, and a Russian immigrant named Viola, so that we could learn subjects with our own special teacher at our own pace.

And it wasn't just in academic achievements. I taught myself to play tennis by banging a ball up against the wall downstairs from our building for hours every day. Our neighborhood was racially mixed without actually being integrated, and the playground on top of the Food City in front of our building was filled with white children and their moms during the day, while a posse of black teenagers took over the place at night. During that dusky hour when the area began to change its identity, I befriended a teenage boy named Paul with whom I regularly played some version of squash. The fact that he was so much stronger really helped my game. But when my mom found out about Paul—who was, she noticed, a *black teenager* and therefore probably on drugs—she somehow dug up the money to pay for tennis lessons at school. There were no more afternoons on the streets after that. It wasn't until I was sent away to summer camp and first confronted the Jappy girls from Long Island, who had hours of private lessons and country club memberships and courts in their back yards, that I began to doubt that I could grow up to be Chris Evert.

It is hard for me to remember a life that was so cocksure, so free of self-doubt, so pure in its certainty. How did all that life-force energy turn so completely into a death wish? How quickly it seemed that my well-developed superego managed to dissolve into buckets of free-flowing, messy id.

You see, until I really cracked up, at ten or eleven or twelve or whenever it was, you most certainly would have described me as, well, as *full of promise*. That term is loaded with irony to me now because I know how false that appearance of promise is. I know how much latent discontent and sorrow that visible determination can mask, but still I am sure that at one time there was a ruddiness in my cheeks, a beaming excitedness in my eyes that suggested so much possibility. I was an astronaut who was going to fly so high, so far beyond the moon, so far beyond the whole wide world.

But then I never had to worry about a crash landing because I never even took off.

2

Secret Life

✳ ✳ ✳

It was like sawdust, the unhappiness: it infiltrated everything, everything was a problem, everything made her cry—school, homework, boyfriends, the future, the lack of future, the uncertainty of future, fear of future, fear in general—but it was so hard to say exactly what the problem was in the first place.

MELANIE THERNSTROM
The Dead Girl

I go to Dr. Isaac's office twice a week, which, I think, if I were a normal eleven-year-old kid I would hate and resent, but being me, I like it fine. He asks me a lot of questions about myself and my life, and being someone who just loves to talk, especially about my problems, I think it is mostly a lot of fun. I can't imagine that we're actually accomplishing anything in these sessions. I mean, I really do believe we might have gotten to the bottom of the root of the mess if such a place existed, but my misery is just too random. Dr. Isaac would occasionally make pronouncements that seemed sensible. He'd say, Because your parents divorced when you were so young and pursued such different lifestyles with such clashing value systems, you have a split foundation, you are a fragmented person. Or he'd say, You're very precocious and very sensitive, and as a result you were extremely attuned to all the terrible things going on around you when you were little, so the damage is surfacing now. Everything he says seems perfectly plausible, but it's all one big *so what*? as far as I'm concerned. I know all this stuff already. For me the problem is what to do about it.

Dr. Isaac is the psychiatrist that the school psychologist recommended to my mother when I started to spend more time hanging out in her office than in the classroom. Or maybe she recommended him after the time Mrs. Edelman, the math teacher who doubled as the girls' basketball coach, found me in the locker room one day wounding my legs with a pack of razor blades while my tape recorder played Patti Smith's *Horses*. Without even bothering to ask what I was doing (though she did ask what I was listening to), Mrs. Edelman dragged me upstairs to the psychologist's office—literally pulled me across the floor by my arm until we got to the elevator that was reserved for teachers only, which made me feel special—and deposited me inside her door, pointing at me as if to say, *Look at this*, as if she were an attorney and I were exhibit A, all the material evidence she needed to make her case. And the point was: This child needs professional help.

I think in exchange for solemnly swearing I would never cut myself again, I got the psychologist, who was called Dr. Bender even though she had only a master's degree, to promise she wouldn't tell my mom about what was wrong with me. About the razors.

I guess the cutting began when I started to spend my lunch period hiding in the girls' locker room, scared to death of everybody around me. I would bring my functional black and silver Panasonic, meant for voice recording and not music, and I would listen intently to the scratchy sound of the tapes I'd accumulated, mostly popular hard rock like Foreigner, which, trashy as it was, sounded like liberation to me. I'd sit there with my tape recorder, eating cottage cheese and pineapples from a stout thermos I brought from home (I was, by this time,

*also certain that I was fat), and it was a peaceful relief from having
to deal with other people, whether they were teachers or friends.*

*Every so often, I would sit in the locker room on the floor,
leaning against the concrete wall while my tape recorder sat on the
bench, and I would fantasize about going back to the person I had
always been. The reverse transformation couldn't be that much of a
leap. I could just try talking to people again. I could get the astonished
look off my face, as if my eyes had just been exposed to a terrible
glare. I could laugh a bit.*

*I would imagine myself doing the things I once did, like playing
tennis. Every so often I would make a decision, first thing in the
morning as I headed out the door for the school bus, that I was going
to be bright-eyed and bushy-tailed that day; I would be friendly, I
would smile, I would raise my hand in math class from time to time.
I remember those days, because I could see how my friends would get
this look of relief on their faces. I would walk toward them, standing
in a huddle in the blue-carpeted hall outside of the classroom, and
they would half expect me to say something like* Everything's plastic, we're all gonna die . . . *and instead I would just say,* Good
morning. *And suddenly, their bodies would relax, their shoulders
would drop comfortably, and sometimes they would even say,* Oh
wow, you're the old Lizzy again, *kind of like a parent who has
finally accepted that his oldest son has become a Shiite Muslim and
is moving to Iran when, suddenly, the kid returns home and announces that he wants to go to law school after all. My friends, and
my mother for that matter, would be relieved to find that I was more
the me they wanted me to be.*

*The trouble was, I thought this alternative persona that I had
adopted was just that: a put-on, a way of getting attention, a way
of being different. And maybe when I first started walking around
talking about plastic and death, maybe then it was an experiment.
But after a while, the alternative me really just was me. Those days
that I tried to be the little girl I was supposed to be drained me. I
went home at night and cried for hours because so many people in*

my life expecting me to be a certain way was too much pressure, as if I'd been held against a wall and interrogated for hours, asked questions I couldn't quite answer any longer.

I remember being in a panic one day at school when I realized that I could not even fake being the old Lizzy anymore. I had, indeed, metamorphosed into this nihilistic, unhappy girl. Just like Gregor Samsa waking up to find he'd become a six-foot-long roach, only in my case, I had invented the monster and now it was over-taking me. This was what I'd come to. This was what I'd be for the rest of my life. Things were bad now and would get worse later. They would. I had not heard the word depression yet, and would not for some time after that, but I felt something very wrong going on. In fact, I felt that I was wrong—my hair was wrong, my face was wrong, my personality was wrong—my God, my choice of flavors at the Häagen-Dazs shop after school was wrong! How could I walk around with such pasty white skin, such dark, doleful eyes, such straight anemic hair, such round hips and such a small cinched waist? How could I let anybody see me this way? How could I expose other people to my person, to this bane to the world? I was one big mistake.

And so, sitting in the locker room, petrified that I was doomed to spend my life hiding from people this way, I took my keys out of my knapsack. On the chain was a sharp nail clipper, which had a nail file attached to it. I rolled down my knee socks (we were required to wear skirts to school) and looked at my bare white legs. I hadn't really started shaving yet, only from time to time because my mother considered me too young, and I looked at the delicate peach fuzz, still soft and untainted. A perfect, clean canvas. So I took the nail file, found its sharp edge, and ran it across my lower leg, watching a red line of blood appear across my skin. I was surprised at how straight the line was and at how easy it was for me to hurt myself this way. It was almost fun. I was always the sort to pick scabs and peel sunburned skin in sheets off my shoulders, always pestering my body. This was just the next step. And how much more satisfying it was to muck up my own body than relying on mosquitoes and walks in *the country among thorny bushes to do it for me. I made a few more scratches, alternating between legs, this time moving the file more quickly, less cautiously.*

I did not, you see, want to kill myself. Not at that time, anyway. But I wanted to know that if need be, if the desperation got so terribly bad, I could inflict harm on my body. And I could. Knowing this gave me a sense of peace and power, so I started cutting up my legs all the time. Hiding the scars from my mother became a sport of its own. I collected razor blades, I bought a Swiss army knife, I became fascinated with the different kinds of sharp edges and the different cutting sensations they produced. I tried out different shapes—squares, triangles, pentagons, even an awkwardly carved heart, with a stab wound at its center, wanting to see if it hurt the way a real broken heart could hurt. I was amazed and pleased to find that it didn't.

Enter Dr. Isaac.

His office is on 40th Street and Second Avenue, a long ride on the M104 from school, so I often have to leave early. I consider this a huge advantage: I hate school. Sometimes I will schedule appointments with him in the middle of the day, telling my mom that there was no other time available, and then I leave school and don't bother to come back. Dr. Isaac asks me about this: Aren't you missing a lot of school lately, Elizabeth? Sometimes I lie to him and say it's a day off, it's some rabbi from the fifteenth century's birthday or something like that, but after a while I figure—I mean, he *is* my therapist—I might as well just tell him I'm cutting. Cutting school, that is.

My truancy is starting to show. My grades fall below B's. I used to practically flagellate myself for getting anything below an A—I mean, an A−was cause for alarm—and now I simply do not care at all. Teachers pull me aside to ask what's wrong. They make themselves available, say things like, If you ever want to talk, I'm here for you. They tell me that they know I can do better than this. My Talmud teacher, Rabbi Gold, takes away the leather-bound copy of *Through the Looking Glass* which I read under my desk during class instead of trying to follow the convoluted rabbinical argument about exactly how big a drop of milk has to be to render an entire pot of meat nonkosher (one sixtieth of the whole is the conclusion, but some disputing parties say one sixty-ninth). After class, he tries to talk to me, though I fade into abstraction. I hear him muttering some words in his vaguely liturgical singsong voice—something like, When one of my most brilliant students can't even tell me what sidrah we're studying today, I know something is wrong—but I just don't care. I feel bad that I've insulted this nice man with my indifference to what he's teaching, but I don't see what I can do about it. I don't care that I don't care, but I do care maybe a little bit about not caring about not caring (if you can follow the convolutions)—but maybe I do feel sorry for all the nice people whose efforts are wasted on a waste case like me. All this just amounts to more grist for the mill of the ill: On top of feeling sad, I also feel guilty.

I explain the same thing to everybody: It all seems pointless in light of the fact that we're all going to die eventually. Why do anything—why wash my hair, why read *Moby Dick*, why fall in love, why sit through six hours of *Nicholas Nickleby*, why care about American intervention in Central America, why spend time trying to get into the right schools, why dance to the music when all of us are just slouching toward the same inevitable conclusion? The shortness of life, I keep saying, makes everything seem pointless when I think about the longness of death. When I look ahead, all I can see is my final demise. And they say, But maybe not for seventy or eighty years. And I say, Maybe you, but me, I'm already gone.

No one seems willing to ask what I mean by that, which

is a good thing because I don't know. It's not that I'm fixing to die any time soon, but my spirit seems to have already retreated to the netherworld, and I figure, Hey, how much longer does my body have? People talk about the way disembodied spirits roam the world with no place to park themselves, but all I can think is that I am a dispirited body, and I'm sure there are plenty of other human mollusk shells roaming around, waiting for some soul to fill them up. At any rate, I don't really explain what I mean when I talk about death, but I am keenly aware that I am frightening people more than a little bit, and I realize that this is the only small delight I get anymore: knowing that others worry, watching them get this sad, discouraged look on their face, like, Shit, bring in the professionals. I take pleasure in the pain I cause others: My life has become a tearjerker movie, and I am glad to be having the calculated effect.

My mother cries when she sees my report card. Ellie, what's happening to you? she asks. She cries some more. *My baby! What's happened to my baby?* She calls Dr. Isaac and asks why he can't make me better faster. She goes to see him, and pretty soon she's so crazy from dealing with me that she's a patient of his too.

By now I have an entire secret life that my mother either doesn't know or doesn't want to know about: Several days a month I wake up in the morning and get dressed to go to school, but instead I take my knapsack and head over to the local McDonald's, drink tea and eat an Egg McMuffin for breakfast, wait until my mother has left for work at 9:00, and then I go back home and get into bed for the rest of the day. Sometimes I go to the New York Public Library on 42nd Street and read old articles about Bruce Springsteen on microfilm. I am particularly proud that I've found the stories from the week of October 5, 1975, when Bruce had appeared on the covers of *Time* and *Newsweek* simultaneously. But mostly I watch the ABC lineup of soap operas, from *All My Children* to *One Life to Live* to *General Hospital*, lying blissfully under the covers in my mother's bed the whole time.

Sometimes I lie in my own bed and listen to music for hours. Always Bruce Springsteen, which is weird, I have to admit, because I'm becoming this really urban punked-out kid, and he is kind of the spokesman of the rumpled, working-class suburbs. But I identify with him so completely that I start to wish I could be a boy in New Jersey. I try to convince my mother that we should move out there, that she should work in a factory or as a waitress in a roadside diner or as a secretary at a storefront insurance office. I want so badly to have my life circumstances match the oppressiveness I feel internally. It all starts to seem ridiculous: After all, Springsteen songs are about getting the hell *out* of the New Jersey grind, and here I am trying to convince my mom that we ought to get *into* it. I'm figuring, if I can just become poor white trash, if I can just get in touch with the blue collar blues, then there'll be a reason why I feel this way. I will be a fucked-up Marxian worker person, alienated from the fruits of my labor. My misery will begin to make sense.

That is all I want in life: for this pain to seem purposeful.

The idea that a girl in private school in Manhattan could have problems worth this kind of trouble seemed impossible to me. The concept of white, middle-class, educated despair just never occurred to me, and listening to rock and roll all day was probably no way to discover it. I didn't know about Joni Mitchell or Djuna Barnes or Virginia Woolf or Frida Kahlo yet. I didn't know there was a proud legacy of women who'd turned overwhelming depression into prodigious art. For me there was just Bruce—and the Clash, the Who, the Jam, the Sex Pistols, all of those punk bands talking about toppling the system in the U.K., which had nothing to do with being so lonesome you could die in the U.S.A.

Maybe I could have picked up a guitar myself and written some rants of my own, but somehow the Upper West Side of Manhattan as a metaphor for lost and embittered youth was not nearly as resonant as Springsteen's songs about hiding in the back streets or riding the Tilt-A-Whirl or the sound of a calliope on the Jersey Shore. Nothing about my life seemed worthy of art or literature or even of just plain life. It seemed too stupid, too girlish, too middle-class. All that was left for me to do was shut down and enter the world of Bruce Springsteen, of music about people from somewhere else, for people doing something else, that would just have to do, because for the moment, for me, there was nothing else.

I think to myself: I have finally gotten so impossible and unpleasant that they will really have to do something to make me better. And then I realize, they think they are doing all they can and it's not working. They have no idea what a bottomless pit of misery I am. They will have to do more and more and more. They think the psychiatrist ought to be enough, they think making the kind of cursory efforts any parents make when their kid is slipping away will be enough, but they don't know how enormous my need is. They don't know how much I will demand of them before I even think about getting better. They do not know that this is not some practice fire drill meant to prepare them for the real inferno, because the real thing is happening right now. All the bells say: too late. *It's much too late and I'm so sure that they are still not listening. They still don't know that they need to do more and more and more, they need to try to get through to me until they haven't slept or eaten or breathed fresh air for days, they need to try until they've died for me. They have to suffer as I have. And even after they've done that, there will still be more. They will have to rearrange the order of the cosmos, they will have to end the cold war, they will have to act like loving, kind adults who care about each other, they will have to cure hunger in Ethiopia and end the sex-slave trade in Thailand and stop torture in Argentina. They will have to do more than they ever thought they could if they want me to stay alive. They have no idea how much energy and exasperation I am willing to suck out of them until I feel better. I will drain them and drown them until they know how little of me there is left even after I've taken everything they've got to give me because I hate them for not knowing.*

While I am unraveling in the slow, tedious manner of a knotted, tangled ball of yarn that's been clawed and twisted and gnarled by a whole bunch of mean, feverish cats, my mom is pretty much refusing to acknowledge that any of this is happening. She's sending me to therapy and all, but she's still taking me along with her to family events like baseball games on Father's Day; she's still sending me to summer camp, drug overdose or no; she's still expecting me to behave myself at the dinner table; she's still treating me like her favorite prop or carry-on accessory. Anyone else can plainly see that it might be better if I were holed up in a hospital, somewhere where it wouldn't seem odd for me to walk out in the middle of *Fast Times at Ridgemont High* to slash up my legs, somewhere where no one would find it weird that every so often I would run out of the room and howl in a state of hysteria while all the normal people would pretend it wasn't happening.

In retrospect, maybe my mother did the right thing: By treating me like a normal kid, like her perfect baby, maybe she kept me from falling down further. After all, by forcing me to participate in real life, she might have prevented me from indulging and wallowing in a depression that might have been even more bottomless and intractable than the one I was experiencing. I have no way of knowing what might have happened had she viewed the situation differently. I'll never know. She was the kind of mother who believed in pulling a Band-Aid off fast, getting over the pain in a snap; but she seemed resigned to let this depression drag on for years, to let this particular bandage come off slowly. Of course, she would never see it that way: She wanted the pain to be over really quickly in this case too, but she seemed to think that ignoring it would make it go away (Band-Aids sometimes do fall off by themselves). So mostly I remember having this nagging, gnawing feeling that I wished she would just let me be as bad as I was. I wished she'd let me sink way down low in front of her, let slide the need to maintain appearances just long enough for me to bottom out and get the kind of help Dr. Isaac was never going to give me. It was as if my therapy sessions with the doctor were one big buffer zone, a dopey palliative that would keep me afloat but would never really allow me to land in the depth of my despair. And I was starting to want to know the worst, I wanted to know how bad it could get.

But she wanted to keep things as good as they could be. We'd always been a team, we'd always been so close, I'd always been her date for the kinds of occasions other women brought their husbands to, I'd always been her best friend— and it seemed that by cracking up I was letting her down. Failing her. I always felt a sense of responsibility toward her— I often felt like the oldest son of a recently widowed woman who is incapable of, say, programming her VCR by herself— and it made me feel extremely restricted in the range of negative emotions I was able to express. I could skip school, I could get lousy grades, I could hide in the girls' locker room for hours, but I could never completely drop out, I could never lose my mind to the point where they'd have to send me away to a loony bin or some place for juvenile defectives because *my mother would not be able to survive such a personal debacle.* She barely wanted to know about the extent of the despair I was able to experience. You should be telling this stuff to Dr. Isaac, she'd say every time I tried to talk to her about my depression. It's not that she was insensitive—sometimes she actually would try to talk to me about why I was like I was—but she just couldn't stand it when I'd explain that nothing at all was wrong, that it was just a matter of everything. She'd want me to be specific: Is this because your father and I don't get along? She'd want me to toss her some solution-oriented problem. She seemed to think I was like a quadratic equation, but the lack of a clear, discernible task to work with made her too crazy.

One night, very late, she walked into my bedroom to find me lying face down on my shag carpet with a set of big, bulbous earphones on, listening to a live bootleg of a Bruce Springsteen tune called "The Promise," and bawling because everything about the desolation of the song seemed so terribly true (the last line was something like "We're gonna take it all, and throw it all away"). She started screaming at me, telling me she couldn't stand any more of this craziness, demanding that I explain to her right now what exactly was wrong. *What what what?* I just sat there, crying, blank, nothing to say, and she kept demanding that I tell her something, and I think in frustration I might have just said, Oh, Ma, you're looking at all the trees, and I'm not even in the forest. And then she went to her room, smoked a cigarette, watched the eleven o'clock news, fell asleep with the blue light of the television still on, feeling completely helpless.

After a while, it was always like this: I'd be lying helpless in my room, she'd be lying helpless in hers, there was nothing we could do to make each other feel better, and the whole apartment seemed stuck in some miserable detente.

Does that make any sense? Is it possible that I didn't collapse, become incapacitated, a nonfunctioning mental case of the catatonic kind, because *my mother wouldn't let me*? I mean, when people just flat out fall apart, when they get into the kind of state where they think they're talking to angels and they sleep barefoot in the park in the middle of winter, it's not as if they *got permission* to be that way. They are that way because they can't help it. Had I been far enough gone, I'd have gone there too. Right?

Maybe. Maybe not. The measure of our mindfulness, the touchstone for sanity in this society, is our level of productivity, our attention to responsibility, our ability to plain and simple hold down a job. If you're still at the point when you're even just barely going through the motions—showing up at work, paying the bills—you are still okay or okay enough. A desire not to acknowledge depression in ourselves or those close to us—better known these days as *denial*, is such a strong urge that plenty of people prefer to think that until you are actually flying out of a window, you don't have a problem. But this does not take into account the socioeconomic factors, the existence of guilt, of a disciplined moral conscience, or in my case, an understanding of my mother's precarious, delicate nature—which placed definite limits on how much rope I had to hang myself. My mother and I had switched roles so often—I helped her pick out boyfriends after the divorce, soaked her cigarettes in water so that she couldn't smoke, or told her, as she sat bawling in the kitchen because she had just lost a job and was scared we'd be broke, that I was sure everything would be all right—and I was afraid to abandon the parental responsibility I felt for her. I knew the limits of the people who were close to me, and in my worst downs, I was ever more attuned to them. Depression gave me extreme perspicacity; rather than skin, it was as if I had only thin gauze bandages to shield me from everything I saw.

My depression did not occur in a vacuum, nor did it eradicate my urge and desire to get better if there was an earthly way to do so. As my mind seemed to slow-drip out of control, I was still able to contain some of the loss, to make use of the geeky A-student discipline I had cultivated over the years. I kept it all within the realm of something happening to a girl who still manages to wear designer jeans, who is still interested in applying purple mascara and turquoise eyeliner before leaving the house in the morning. I made myself presentably pretty each day just in case the man of my dreams happened to be waiting on the sidewalk outside of Manhattan Day School, all set to carry me away from the geography of my depression, kind of the way Sam Shepard carries off Jessica Lange at the beginning of the movie *Frances*, or the way he remains in love with her thirty years later, after she's had a full frontal lobotomy.

And so, at age twelve, with more and more frequency, I'd find myself sitting inside McDonald's early in the morning eating my Egg McMuffin, my attention fixed on some of the hard luck cases sitting nearby in the orange and red seats, muttering to themselves, wearing clothes that were filthy, smelling from sleeping on the sidewalks and drinking too much Colt 45, and I contemplated the difference and the distance between them and me. How far to go before I, or anyone like me, fell into such a derelict, dehumanized place? Did you have to survive Vietnam (so many of the panhandlers on the subways seemed to be veterans) or did it take poverty, chemical dependency, severe mental illness, and long years in state institutions for this to happen? I would never know.

I must have understood that my material circumstances were such that I alone could keep myself from falling. I mean, if I were a rich kid with stable, self-sufficient parents whom I thought I could trust to attend to themselves and to me, and I were heading for a tailspin, I might feel free to let myself free-fall, knowing that someone else would provide a bottom upon which I might eventually bottom out. But what if you are the only resting point you know of? What if you are absolute zero? What if only you can catch yourself?

Mr. Grubman, the very strange science teacher who wears a beret and black turtlenecks every day like a beatnik, keeps me after class because he says my behavior is disruptive. I can't imagine what he means: I'm not one of those kids who sets all the frogs free before we can dissect them, and anyway what we're mostly doing in class is squeezing sour milk through cheesecloth as a way to help us understand the phenomena of everyday life. He's just the latest in a long series of science teachers, maybe the fourth this year, so it's hard for me to take him seriously. He's probably not the one who will be giving me a grade in the end because he too will surely be replaced, and anyway grades don't matter to me anymore because there's no future.

At any rate, Mr. Grubman doesn't seem to want to talk to me about much. He says, You seem like maybe you're too intense for this world, and I wonder where he's getting that from. He barely knows me. It sounds like he's suggesting I kill myself.

He keeps me in the science lab for hours. I miss a bunch of classes, and even eat my lunch, cottage cheese with pine-apples in a thermos as usual, in his classroom. After a while I have no idea what he wants from me, I am only glad that I don't have to sit through math and English or play kickball during gym because he is keeping me here as a punishment. He asks me lots of questions that I don't know the answers to. He asks, So are you one of those girls who likes fast guys with fast cars?

I don't say what I am really thinking, which is that I'm only twelve so I don't know and in New York no one drives anyway. Instead, I just say, Yes, yes I do.

It seems like the right answer.

Boys are one interest of mine that never really goes away, though to little avail. None of the guys I go to school with notice me. I'm not even on their lists of alternatives after all the girls with names like Jennifer and Alison and Nicole don't work out. It's not that I'm unattractive—I think that maybe I'm even pretty, but my look appeals to an entirely different demographic group. I have cultivated a certain shaggy paleness, I have that boozy and bruise-eyed Chrissie Hynde look, so I end up attracting older guys who are used to women who aren't bright and cheery. Or else I pick up these rocker types, like the guy in the heavy metal band who works at a store called the World Import at the Bergen Mall, where I sometimes go when I cut school. Or the man who gave me his business card during a riot at a Clash concert who takes me to lunch every so often. Or the twenty-three-year-old son of the owner of Camp Tagola, who is actually in law school and is very straight and decent, but still is attracted enough to me that it becomes kind of a scandal around camp and the head counselor tells us both that we have to stop taking walks together or sitting side by side while we watch *Stalag 17*. But nothing much ever happens with any of these men. It's all just so much lunch, so many walks and talks, because I'm too young and they're too old so they feel stupid. I find myself praying, wishing, hoping that God could just give me whatever it is that makes girls attractive to boys my age.

And then one day I meet my friend's older brother, a Springsteen fan who's a senior in high school. We talk about Bruce all the time, and he thinks it's amazing that I'm not like all his sister's other friends who are into Shaun Cassidy and Andy Gibb. I get such a crush on him—his name is Abel—and after a while I'm going to my friend's house to see him more than to visit her. I feel this strange affinity, like maybe he might like me too, and one night when we're watching TV in the den with the whole family—it's Tuesday night, so I bet it was *Happy Days* or *Laverne and Shirley*—and I am sitting under an afghan quilt to keep warm, I feel his hand reach underneath the blanket, up my legs, into my panties. I don't try to stop him, I do nothing at all but sit there and take in the sensation because it feels good, it is the only thing that has felt nice to me at all in so many months, maybe even years. I have never had a feeling quite like this before, haven't even come close to the strange electricity that seems to be spinning in my stomach and then just below, and below and below and below. And I can't imagine what I've done to deserve anything so nice.

And I feel blessed. I feel that if God has given me this capacity for pleasure, then there must be hope. So I start sneaking into Abel's bedroom in the middle of the night whenever I sleep over at their house, start wishing he could do to me what he does to me all the time because I never knew my body had such a capacity for joy. I learn to touch him too. With my fingers, my hands, my mouth. I am surprised to discover that I have the facility, in all my sadness, not only to receive but to give a bit of this life force.

This physical contact brings me such happiness that I want to tell everybody I know about it, I want to walk up to women in the streets and tell them about this thing I've discovered, as if only I am privy to it. I want to give blowjobs to guys I see here and there, wondering if they will respond the way Abel does, or is it just something unique to him. I want to let Dr. Isaac know this little secret of mine, but I can't say a word to a soul. Everyone will think it's sick, will think I am being molested because he's seventeen and I'm only twelve. No one will ever believe that this is the only good thing in my life.

So when Mr. Grubman bothers me with all his questions—his strange, salacious questions—I think to myself that maybe I should tell him my secret. But then I don't, don't dare. I am somehow afraid of how weird he is, afraid that he will turn me in and then they will send me away, lock me up in a prison for unchaste girls. I am scared that they will throw me into an institution not because I am depressed and need help, but because I am a girl, a good girl in my own way, and still I am capable of such crazy lust.

That summer, I am just thirteen, everything sucks and I am stuck at camp wondering about the Olympics. One day right after clean-up period, right after our beds have been inspected for hospital corners and our cubbies have been checked to make sure all the Archie comics are piled neatly, I sit on the porch of my bunk listening to Bruce Springsteen's first album. Paris, a girl I also go to school with, comes outside to sit with me. Paris is, I guess, what I would call a friend. I've known her since kindergarten, and like everyone else who's been in my life for a while, she's just kind of waiting for me to snap out of this funk so that we can have play dates and polish our nails in baby pink like we used to do when we were seven. She lives across the street from me so we still walk home from school together sometimes, which can't be any fun for her because all I want to talk about is the oncoming apocalypse in my brain.

Paris tries to be understanding. I don't make this process very easy for people. After weeks of haranguing the girls in my bunk about the genius of Bruce Springsteen, when they finally say that they're getting to like him, when they ask to borrow tapes or make requests to hear *Born to Run*, I just start yelling that they're all a bunch of unoriginal copycats and Bruce belongs to me alone. I make them swear that if they ever meet anyone new and claim to like any Springsteen songs, they'll remember to footnote me. And they all throw up their hands and say, Look, we're trying. So Paris comes and sits down beside me, and I make her a little nervous when

I tell her that she's got to listen to this song called "For You." She's afraid I'll be cross if she doesn't like it, or—even worse—that I'll be really furious if she does. I explain that the song is about a girl just like me who kills herself. We listen to the first verse, to the cryptic lines about a girl's fading presence, about "barroom eyes shine vacancy," about someone whose grip on life is so vague that to see her you have to look hard.

That's me, I say to Paris. I'm the girl who is lost in space, the girl who is disappearing always, forever fading away and receding farther and farther into the background. Just like the Cheshire cat, someday I will suddenly leave, but the artificial warmth of my smile, that phony, clownish curve, the kind you see on miserably sad people and villains in Disney movies, will remain behind as an ironic remnant. I am the girl you see in the photograph from some party someplace or some picnic in the park, the one who looks so very vibrant and shimmery, but who is in fact soon going to be gone. When you look at that picture again, I want to assure you, *I will no longer be there*. I will be erased from history, like a traitor in the Soviet Union. Because with every day that goes by, I feel myself becoming more and more invisible, getting covered over more thickly with darkness, coats and coats of darkness that are going to suffocate me in the sweltering heat of the summer sun that I can't even see anymore, even though I can feel it burn.

Imagine, I suggest to Paris, only knowing that the sun is shining because you feel the ache of its awful heat and not because you know the joy of its light. Imagine being always in the dark.

I am going on and on this way to Paris, who is still uneasy, and is not quite sure what to say. You know, I continue, I'd be just like the girl in the song except for one thing. One thing. And that's that he says she's all he ever wanted.

He loves her so much. The whole song is about how he's come to take her to the hospital, to rescue her from suicide.

I start, as if on cue, to cry. I am so caught up in the idea that nobody would actually try to save me if I were to slit my wrists or hang myself from one of the rafters in the bunk. I can't believe anyone might care enough to try to keep me alive. And then I realize that, yes, of course they would, but only because it is the thing to do. It's not about true caring. It's about not wanting to live with the guilt, the insult, the ugly knowledge that a suicide took place and you did nothing. Once I make a suicidal gesture, then everyone indeed will come running because my problems leave the realm of the difficult, workaday, let's-talk-it-through stuff and I become an actual medical emergency. I will qualify as a trauma case that Aetna or MetLife, or whichever insurance carrier I've got, will actually cover. They'll pump my stomach, stitch my wrists, apply cold packs to the bruises on my neck, do whatever it is they have to do to keep me alive—and then the heavy-duty, institutional-size mental health professionals take over.

But day after day of depression, the kind that doesn't seem to merit carting me off to a hospital but allows me to sit here on this stoop in summer camp as if I were normal, day after day wearing down everybody who gets near me. My behavior seems, somehow, not acute enough for them to know what to do with me, though I'm just enough of a mess to be driving everyone around me crazy.

I cry some more and go on and on about how nice it must be to have someone so in love with you they'd sing about the day you died. Paris opens her mouth, probably to say something about how people would like to help, people would like to let me know they care, they just don't know what to do, but I shut her up. I don't want to hear the company line right now. And if anyone ever loved me enough to write such a beautiful song about me, you know I wouldn't kill myself, I continue. In the end I have to think the girl in "For You" is totally crazy because she decided to die when there was so much love for her right here on earth.

Yes, Paris says, talking to me only to offer the comfort of a human voice, not because she can say anything that will make a difference. I see what you mean.

Oh, Paris. I cry some more. No one is ever going to love me that way because I'm so awful and all I ever do is cry and get depressed.

If I were another person, I go on, *I* wouldn't want to deal with me. I *don't* want to deal with me. It's so hopeless. I want out of this life. I really do. I keep thinking that if I could just get a grip on myself, I could be all right again. I keep thinking that I'm driving myself crazy, but I swear, I swear to God, I have no control. It's so awful. It's like demons have taken over my mind. And nobody believes me. Everybody thinks I could be better if I wanted to. But I can't be the old Lizzy anymore. I can't be myself anymore. I mean, actually, I am being myself right now and it's so horrible.

Paris just puts her arms around me and hugs me. Lizzy, everyone likes you fine just the way you are, she says, because that's what people say in these situations.

I sit there with my face in my hands as if to catch my head, to keep it from falling off and rolling across girls' campus like a soccer ball that someone might kick by accident.

3

Love Kills

✳ ✳ ✳

When I think of all the things he did because he loved me—what people visit on each other out of something like love. It's enough for all the world's woe. You don't even need hate to have a perfectly miserable time.

RICHARD BAUSCH
Mr. Field's Daughter

By the time I made it to eighth grade, my parents were ready to kill each other. For the first time since their divorce, they had to talk pretty regularly about what to do with me. These were hopeless and frustrating discussions, no doubt, because every little thing always seemed to make me worse. I was like an already overspiced stew, and all the chefs adding all their condiments were only making it more foggy and muddled and bad.

And my parents were a disastrous pairing for getting anything much accomplished. Here were two people who had barely spoken for ten years, just passing each other in the vestibule as they passed me back and forth between them, and now they were suddenly in constant contact, mostly yelling and fighting violently on the phone late at night. I would hear my mother's voice as I lay, not sleeping, not even trying to sleep, in my bedroom. And sometimes, when I was deep in a slumber, the sound of them shouting in the other room would invade my dreams like a foreign army. My mother's end turned up loud and clear while my father's side was left to the vivid realm of imagination. They argued about whether Dr. Isaac was right for me, about who would pay for what, and, above all, whose fault it was that I was so messed up. They unearthed old controversies, and it was clear that if their problems had ever been buried, it was a very shallow and degraded grave. The pettiness was horrific: My father would complain that when I needed braces my mother managed to pick the most expensive, crooked, shyster of an orthodontist; my mother retorted that his insurance covered ninety percent of it anyway so what did he care. He accused her of always wanting to spend more than either of them had so that I could go to private schools and wear pretty clothes; she would scream that if he'd prefer, I could just as easily go to some horrible public school in Queens, where he lived at the time, and take up with kids who had poor elocution and never went to Bach recitals or exhibits at the Met. Then all she could say was that it was lucky for me that she was the custodial parent. He said she was living in a dream world; she said he was living in a dream world.

Though I could not hear his exact words, I know he must have accused her of being a lousy mother, which would trigger more screaming on her end; this allegation was the same as telling my mom that her whole life was worthless, that she wasn't even good at the one thing she was supposed to be good at. Her response was always the same: Donald, she would yell, I have had to raise our daughter all by myself with almost no help from you. I am a saint, I am. You never took her on vacations. You never took her on weekends. It's all been left to me and I think I've done a pretty good job, thanks not at all to you.

And then the phone would slam and there would be silence followed by her wailing. The sound of her cry was so scary it was as if she were part of the chorus in a Greek tragedy and this was the big funeral scene—and I would think: I am more trouble than I'm worth.

Their belligerence had arrived about a decade late. The procedure of their separation and divorce had been a relatively peaceful one: There was so little money or property to argue about, save for some good china and some bad Jose Feliciano records, that they never even bothered to get separate attorneys; they just had my mother's lawyer-cousin draw up the papers. My mother got custody, my father didn't even fully use his visitation rights, and the combined amount of alimony and child support that he had to pay was fixed at a weekly sum of less than seventy-five dollars. They had such a straightforward and uncomplicated relationship for so many years, or at least so it had seemed, that it was astonishing to watch as my depression became a catalyst for them to address all the mutual rage that they had been sublimating.

When they started doing battle night after night, I remember thinking that something was really wrong here because last I checked, *I* was the one who was supposed to have the problems. They were ostensibly arguing about what would be the best method of treatment for me, but in the meantime, as they lay screaming, I just hid in my room languishing in an increasingly morose state. Occasionally, in an effort to upset my mother, my father would refuse to process my psychiatrist bills through his insurance plan, not realizing that she wasn't going to suffer without the therapy—*I* was. Everything had gotten so damned out of focus. Instead of feeling like a kid whose parents *were* divorced, I felt like a kid whose parents *should* get divorced.

Here was this thing called depression that was not definable in any sort of concrete way (was it bigger than a breadbox? smaller than an armoire? animal, vegetable, or mineral?) that had simply taken up residence in my mind—a mirage, a vision, a hallucination—and yet it was creeping into the lives of everyone who was close to me, ruining them all as I was ruined myself. If it were a pestilence, like the roaches that used to creep around the kitchen of our apartment, we could have called an exterminator; if it were a fire, we could have turned an extinguisher on it; my God, even if it were something simple like having trouble with quadratic equations in algebra class, there were tutors who could have taught me about 2ab or 3^2 or how to mix numbers and letters so they are just right. But this was just madness. I mean, I wasn't an alcoholic, an anorexic, a bulimic, or a drug addict. We couldn't blame this all on booze or food or vomit or thinness or needles and the damage done. My parents could argue until late into the night about what to do about *this*—this thing— but they were basically bickering about something that in measurable terms did not exist.

I found myself *wishing* for a real ailment, found myself longing to be a junkie or a cokehead or something—something real. If it were only a matter of keeping me away from my bad habits, how much easier it all would be. I know now, of course, that alcohol and drugs also mask a type of depression that is not so very different from my own, but getting help for substance abuse can be reduced to the deceptively simple focus of *keeping away from the dope*. But what does getting help with depression mean? Learning to keep away from your own mind? Wouldn't it be a whole lot easier to get rid of Jack Daniel's than Elizabeth Wurtzel?

Around that time, John and Mackenzie Phillips had just gone through rehab to kick their coke habits, and it seemed that every week one or the other of them was on the cover of *People*: Mackenzie because she lost her job on the TV series *One Day at a Time* and married the record producer Peter Asher, who supposedly supplied her with blow; and John because he was going to put the Mamas and the Papas back together now that he was sober. I carefully read about their lives as drug addicts, which seemed to beat the hell out of being depressed like me. For one thing, people who did self-destructive things like drive a BMW into a tree got lots of attention, and for another, they got to be rescued.

Rescued. That's what it looked like to me. Drug addicts had the crutch of a tangible problem—they needed to get sober—so there were places they could be carted off to for help. There were Hazelden and St. Mary's and the Betty Ford Center and the whole state of Minnesota to go to for recovery. Somehow, I got it in my head that rehab was like a conveyor belt that you rode for twenty-eight days or twenty months or however long it took to get better. Then you were pushed off the assembly line all fresh and spanking new, ready to start all over again.

Obviously, this is a prison house fantasy of the life of addiction. Many people go through rehab several times and still don't recover, but it was certainly true that there were many outlets and much alarmist behavior you could indulge in if you developed a nasty drug problem. I, on the other hand, had taken a small overdose of pills and scarred my legs with razor blades, and still no one seemed to be rescuing me. Because, on paper, there was no actual problem. If I had a heroin habit, you can bet my parents would have checked me in faster than it takes a junkie to jiggle blood in a syringe. If I were on drugs, they'd have stuck me in a hospital, where my behavior would be monitored all the time by counselors and doctors, and I'd get to meet other cool drug addicts who were getting clean, so I'd never be lonely. After rehab, I could spend the rest of my life going to Alcoholics Anonymous or Narcotics Anonymous meetings and hanging out with other recovered drug abusers with problems just like mine.

All those celebrity stories about drug abuse were meant to be a caveat to the youth of America, morality tales that were supposed to teach you to Just Say No. But it seemed to me that if I could get hooked on some drug, anything was possible. I'd make new friends. I'd have a real problem. I'd be able to walk into a church basement full of fellow sufferers, and have them all say, Welcome to our nightmare! We understand! Here are our phone numbers, call any time you feel you're slipping because we're here for you.

Here for you: I could not imagine anyone ever being here for me.

Depression was the loneliest fucking thing on earth. There were no halfway houses for depressives, no Depression Anonymous meetings that I knew of. Yes, of course, there were mental hospitals like McLean and Bellevue and Payne Whitney and the Menninger Clinic, but I couldn't hope to end up in one of those places unless I made a suicide attempt serious enough to warrant oxygen or stitches or a stomach pump. Until then, I would remain woefully undertreated by a Manhattan psychiatrist who could offer only a little bit of help amid the chaos of my home life. I used to wish—to pray to God for the courage and strength—that I'd have the guts not to get better, but to slit my wrists and get a whole lot worse so that I could land in some mental ward, where real help might have been possible.

As far as individual therapy went, it's hard for me now to evaluate Dr. Isaac's ability because he spent so much time off in the referee's corner, trying to keep my parents at bay. Since then I have had many more therapists—nine to date—whom I can assess more solidly for their touch and technique. Diana Sterling, M.D., was the only thing standing between me and suicide; later, there would be the idiots like Peter Eichman, Ph.D., a psychologist I saw my freshman year of college who wanted to talk more about the time I arrived at my appointment than about the business at hand. But Dr. Isaac's job was grounded so solidly in crisis management that there is no way for me to judge the work we did together. He was an odd man, with an air of studied casualness: He wore running shoes with his suits and ties, even before the New York City transit strike. But in the midst of his mellow dude approach, Dr. Isaac was also one of those typical self-promoting New York professionals who would happily boast about his many celebrity clients. During one of my long ramblings about Bruce Springsteen or rock and roll as salvation, he would interject that he had once treated Patti Smith, a singer whom I idolized, when she was in a mental hospital. Did I know that he had been the doctor who had examined Mark David Chapman when he was admitted to the psychiatric ward after assassinating John Lennon? Did I know the recently deposed president of NBC was one of his patients? And I would think to myself, I must be really far gone to be worthy of the same therapist as Patti Smith, who after all had cohabited with Sam Shepard and had all of her album portraits taken by Robert Mapplethorpe. But I'd still be left wondering, What's in it for me? Is this therapy or dinner at Elaine's?

As for the family counseling sessions, whatever therapeutic potential our visits with Dr. Isaac might have had were derailed by the manipulations of all three of us trying to get him to make our disastrous little triangle work a bit better, to make it more equilateral than isosceles, or altogether less of a triangle and more of a happy circle. But it was an impossible task. Without a concerted, united effort on the part of the parents, a withdrawn child is not likely to emerge and return to health (although that's a bit like saying the only thing you hate about rain is that it's wet, because unhappy children are often the result of fractured home lives). After a while, Dr. Isaac seemed to resign himself to the idea that he could not truly help me to get better, so the best he could do was just prevent my sinking even lower. Like everything else in my life, our biweekly visits were just a Band-Aid, a small buffer zone full of social prattle and practical advice, but getting down to the bone and the skin and the eyes and the teeth was not in the offing.

In the midst of all this, my mom had pretty much turned Dr. Isaac into her guru, so there was no way I could discuss my misgivings about him with her, and my dad was uncharacteristically thrilled to fill up the power vacuum left by my mom's inability to deal with most of what was happening with me. He liked, almost relished, reading my bad, depressing, adolescent poetry, much of which went something like "I have been encompassed by the night / As its curtain of darkness has wound me in its threads . . ." My mom wasn't interested in my miserable writing, and she just couldn't look at it without feeling awful herself. While she was able to continue competently as a parent on all the usual material fronts—she fed me, she gave me a bed to sleep in, she theoretically sent me to school—she was completely dense about my emotional life. She just didn't want to know about it, had pretty much decided this was a job for the professionals. On the other hand, my father loved chatting with me about how awful the whole world was because he basically agreed. After a while, he was the only one of them I really talked to, and because I was in a vulnerable enough state to believe pretty much whatever loony theories anyone wanted to toss my way, my father came damn close to convincing me that my mother was the sole party responsible for all the ills that beset me. He'd tell me that she sent me to these repressive Jewish schools, she shut him out from being an active parent, and in my desperation to find a locus of blame for all my pain, I'd sometimes think he was right.

Occasionally, my mother would complain that my dad and I were ganging up on her: like the time he enrolled me in guitar lessons and then told her that she was supposed to pay for it because he gave her child support for things like that, or the time he brought me to consultations with a bunch of possible replacements for Dr. Isaac without telling her. She'd yell at me and get furious and say stuff like, Where was he through your whole childhood? He slept through it all and now he's trying to steal you away. He's brainwashing you. Then my mother would spend hours crying on the phone to her sister, who would then have me out to her house on Long Island for a few days so that my mom and I could cool off. Sometimes I would admit to my aunt that I knew deep down that my dad was only taking advantage of my discontent to enrage my mother, but I was happy to take whatever relief from my depression he cared to contribute. I had no scruples: I would do *anything* if it meant I might feel better, even if it made my mom miserable.

Of course, to my mother the most bothersome part of my father's renewed interest in me was the emptiness of his gestures. He could be good to talk to sometimes, but his actual efforts on my behalf added up to a whole lot of nothing. Every time I realized how little he would actually do for me as a father, how indifferent he was to parenting basics like buying me clothes or getting me to school on time or running me over to dance class, my misery was compounded. I could see that he might have understood me better than my mom did, but he really didn't love me as devotedly. He simply liked me more at that point because I had, in all my despair, become rather interesting to him. While he snoozed and napped and zoned out through my childhood, never much excited by my verbal precocity at six, never much taken with my guileless foolishness at nine, he was thoroughly intrigued with the suicidally depressed teenager I had become.

My mother, on the other hand, didn't find it interesting at all: She mourned as she watched me become a morbid, blue stranger who slept in the bed that her child once occupied. One night, in the midst of all these battles, I remember going into my mother's bedroom to kiss her good night. She was lying under her burgundy duvet in her shiny pink nylon nightgown while the independent network news blared from the television. I approached the bed and looked down at her lying there, so small and gentle. Her black hair was twisted around her head, her dark eyes were puffy, coated with the baby oil that she used to remove her make-up, and her dark olive skin, which always made her look as if she'd just gotten a tan in the French Riviera, stretched over her high cheek-bones and sharp nose like a painted canvas. Why had I not gotten her looks, her Mediterranean coloring, her sharply etched features, her huge dark bedroom eyes that slanted just right? Why did I look so much more like my father's family, pale, fleshy, with droopy eyes that always looked lazy, indi-vidual features that tended to fade and blend as if they were as compromised and uncertain as all of our personalities? I remembered a Polaroid of my mother that was taken when she worked at Macy's, with her long black hair and thick bangs separated by a wide headband. She looked just as beau-tiful to me now, although her face had hardened and tough-ened. Age had taken away what little frivolity her arch features had once possessed. But somehow that night, lying in bed, she was all softness and delicacy, a fragile rumble doll.

But I knew she could just as easily snap at me for no apparent reason, and her gaze could turn instantly from loving to harsh. She was that mercurial, especially then, especially since she could not deal with my depression. But as angry as she might sometimes get, as loud as she would yell, and as irrationally as she would rant, in the end she was the parent I could count on. If she and I had a disagreement that was so bad that we didn't talk to each other for days, I could still be certain that dinner would be on the table each evening, that my tuition would be paid, that my clothes would be ironed.

She was my mother and that was that. I could never be so certain about my father. When I would run away from home and spend a night in the shag-carpeted attached house my dad and stepmother had recently moved into in Westchester, using the bathroom soap—we're talking a supermarket brand like Tone, nothing fancy—without asking permission first would throw the whole household into paroxysms. My presence was that strange to them.

Our family life was like the King Solomon story in the Bible, with two women both claiming to be the biological mother of one infant. Like the true mother who would relinquish her right to keep the baby before letting the king cut it in half, I could be certain that my mother would weep for my life and give anything to keep me in one piece, but my father, well, I'm not so sure. He's like me, always compromising, always throwing up his hands, never quite certain of the righteousness of his cause. It would have been just like him to tiredly exclaim, *Tear the child apart*, which is what was happening anyway.

What made my life different from the parable is that both of my parents did have claims. And in order to remain whole, I needed both of them, but that seemed not to be an option. Something inside me was not just depressed but dividing, cracking, splintering, pulling me back and forth between my two parents, and occasionally I wished I could walk through a picture window and have the sharp, broken shards slash me to ribbons so I would finally look like I felt.

Can divorce possibly work when a child is involved? I know that these days a small industry of marriage counselors and divorce therapists devote themselves to easing the process of parental separation for the sake of the children, and I know that all these people are just trying to help, trying to arrange things so that as long as we're stuck in Alaska we might as well have a good warm coat to wear. But can this situation ever really be all right?

Any breakup, even of a brief romance, is rife with potential for all kinds of emotional rampages. So how can we possibly be so pragmatic and realistic and eerily, creepily sane as to ask a couple going through a divorce to try to check their feelings and behave themselves and cooperate and be nice for the sake of the children? Of all the odd demands that modern life makes on humanity, the most difficult may be not only its insistence that we comfortably spend our adult lives going from one situation of serial monogamy to another, but its expectation that we get along, maintain friendships, share parental duties, and in some cases even attend the second and third weddings of our exes. It asks that we pretend that heartbreak is a minor inconvenience that can be overcome with just the right amount of psycholanguage, with just a few repetitions of the mantra for the sake of the children.

I occasionally find myself respecting my parents for making no show of such civility, of not even staging amicability for my sake at my worst moments. I know it would have been better for me had they managed to do that, but I might have been just as distressed by the hypocrisy, the false smiles, the feigned friendliness.

Often during those thirteen-year-old days, I would talk to my father late into the night, drearily rambling about the blackness of it all but sometimes telling him I hated my mother because sometimes I thought I did. I would drag the phone on its long extension cord from my mother's bedroom to the narrow corridor leading to my room and I would speak to him in a whispered hush about my dismal life. Of course, this drove my mother crazy. So when I got off the phone, to make her feel better I'd tell her that Daddy really didn't care about me at all. I'd tell my mom that I hated my dad, which seemed to satisfy her for a little while, long enough for her to seem okay until the next time she found me talking to him in conspiratorial tones about needing to get away from Dr. Isaac, and then she'd cry all over again, telling me that my loyalty to my fa-

ther, my turncoat ways, were making her so sick she was bleeding internally.

One of these nights, she'd threaten, I'm going to be so sick that you're going to have to take me to the emergency room because of the blood, but you'll be too busy complaining about me to your father to even notice, and I will die and then how will you feel?

And then how would I feel? I could never answer straight, I'd just cry and hug her, and let my head fall against her collarbone and say, I don't want this, I don't mean for this, why can't everyone just get along?

In the proper fashion of divorced mothers, during her sane, lucid moments my mother would, of course, pay lip service to the idea that I ought to have a relationship with my father. Everybody needs and deserves a mommy and a daddy. In reality, she didn't want me to get too close to him. She wanted him around, but only in his rightful, Saturday-afternoon place. And who could blame her? How could my mom tell me, whom she loved more than anyone else in the world, that she wanted me to have a good relationship with my father, whom she hated more than anyone else on earth, and not get found out? Ditto my dad.

It is no surprise that a generation of children of divorce have grown into a world of extended adolescence in which so many of them have slept with one another and remained friends, have put the conflicts of sundered relationships aside for the sake of maintaining a coherent life. Divorce has taught us how to sleep with friends, sleep with enemies, and then act like it's all perfectly normal in the morning. Sometimes I have to admire my parents for being so psychologically unenlightened, for avoiding self-help books with titles like I'm O.K., You're O.K., for choosing—or rather, not choosing, but simply instinctually acting—to be true to their own untrammeled, unfettered, unresolved, and unexamined emotional immaturity. Every so often, they would try to put on a face of mutual concern, telling me that their feelings for each other shouldn't affect me, but it always rang false, like putting an elephant in the middle of our cramped, poorly lit living room and trying to suggest that I ignore the

beast, that he would be tame and well behaved, that we could just
live and work around him. I admired the fact that rather than trying
to do what was right in a situation that was so obviously wrong, they
did what came naturally.

We went to Alaska and we froze to death.

I went to camp for five years in a row, a different one each
year, a different setup in a different rural town in the Poconos
or the Catskills or the Berkshires or wherever I could enroll
at a discount rate. And the funny thing is, after my mother
had sent me off to these places that I thought were so lonesome and horrible, instead of hating her for it, I just spent all
summer missing her. All my waking and sleeping energy was
devoted to missing my rather minimal, unstable home. Starting on June 28, or whatever day it was that I got to camp,
until I'd come home on August 24 or so, I would devote
myself fully to the task of getting back home, never even
achieving a brief reprieve.

I'd spend hours each day writing my mom letters,
calling her on the phone, making sure that she'd know exactly where and when to pick me up at the bus when it
was time to return. I would run to the camp's administra-
tive offices to make sure that notices about the return trip
would be sent to my mother so that she'd know where to
find me. I'd extract promises that she'd arrive one or two
hours early. I'd call even my dad and get him to promise
to come at least a half hour before the estimated time of
arrival. I'd talk to the head counselor and express my concern that I might be put on a bus to New Jersey or Long
Island and somehow end up in the wrong place and never
find my way back home. I would ask other New Yorkers
in my bunk if I could go home with them if my mother
failed to materialize at the bus stop. I would call grandparents, aunts, uncles, and babysitters (always collect) to find

out where they would be on August 24, just in case my parents didn't come to get me. Instead of discovering the virtues of tennis and volleyball, of braiding lanyards and weaving potholders, I would spend the full eight weeks of my summer planning for my two-hour trip back home.

Sometimes, even now, when it rains in the summer—the kind of cold, dreary downpour that they're always referring to in blues songs, the kind that makes it feel like autumn or even winter in July—I experience déjà vu, and can feel my head fog over, feel my whole body tense, as I remember the rainy days at camp, those dark, depressing days when the rain came down like blows, when I walked around in my yellow slicker feeling chilled and bruised and battered, wondering what I had done wrong to make my parents banish me. What had I done to deserve this and how could I undo it?

I was such a good kid, I really was. I didn't need anyone to entertain me, I was so resourceful. Left alone I would have probably read the collected works of Tolstoy, or at least Tolkien. I might have sketched on my pad or written another one of the children's books about animals I had started turning out regularly at age five. By God, I was genuinely happy being alone. Which is, I'm sure, the exact reason that I was sent to sleepaway camp and forced to deal with other kids my age: This was yet another bid at making me normal.

I can't get away from the suspicion that it all went wrong at summer camp, that my exile began back then, that my spirit broke—and broke and broke and broke—a little bit more with each passing summer. Everything ended for me at camp. I stopped writing my books, stopped collecting grasshoppers, stopped feeling pretty, stopped wanting to know what makes lightning and rainbows and tsunami winds if it isn't God, stopped wanting to know if there was a God, stopped asking questions that all the adults were too tired to answer anyway, stopped wanting to want anything at all anymore, knowing for sure that I could never have it, that I'd been expelled from that place where possibility still existed.

It doesn't matter how many years go by, how much therapy I embark on, how much I try to achieve that elusive thing known as perspective, which is supposed to put all past wrongs into their rightful and diminished place, that happy place where all the talk is of lessons learned and inner peace. No one will ever understand the potency of my memories, which are so solid and vivid that I don't need a psychiatrist to tell me they are driving me crazy. My subconscious has not buried them, my superego has not restrained them. They are front and center, they are going on right now. And what I feel as I think of summer camp is completely ugly: *I want to kill my parents for doing this to me! I want to hack them to death for this because I was the best little girl in the world and instead of making me feel good about all the things that were good about me, they sent me away and I never really found my way back home! I was special! I had promise! And instead they threw me away and tried to make me ordinary! They threw me away with a bunch of normal kids who thought I was strange and made me feel strange until I became strange! And after all these years, I still despise them for doing this to me!*

The tears come down, not like rain, but like blows.

Homesickness is just a state of mind for me. I'm always missing someone or someplace or something, I'm always trying to get back to some imaginary somewhere. My life has been one long longing.

By the time I go off to Camp Seneca Lake for my fifth and final summer, everything is pandemonium. All I remember are snatches of this and flashes of that chaotic moment. Crying to my father on the phone; my mother crying in the other room on her bed, smoking a cigarette; my father asking me to put my mother on the phone; my mother refusing and then consenting and then crying and pleading with him, asking why he is interfering with the relationship that she and I have. She cries some more. I cry some. My mother and I, each of us in our respective rooms, crying. And yelling. And making up. And hugging and kissing and crying some more because we swear we're never going to let Daddy come between us again. And then, sure enough, Daddy comes between us when Mommy isn't busy coming between me and Daddy. That's sort of how it went in those days. I was always betraying one of them with the other. As if this were a love triangle. Which, of course, it was.

My mother starts to scream and cry about everything I do. When I get a second hole pierced in my ear, she goes nuts and I have to go stay with her sister for a few days. When she sees me talking to my father on the telephone in that conspiratorial tone, the one she recognizes so well without even hearing a word I'm saying, she retreats to her room, to her pack of Gauloises, and goes from numb to hysterical and back again. She calls her sister a lot. She tells me I am upsetting her so much that the internal bleeding is starting to get real bad, that soon I will drive her to an early grave. I tell her that I don't want to make her sad, I just want a relationship with my father and I don't want one with Dr. Isaac. She says that Dr. Isaac saved my life and that Daddy is interfering with the therapeutic process.

And then I say, Well, I disagree.

My dad refuses to pay Dr. Isaac's bills even though insurance covers almost all of it, so my mother has to find the money from the pittance she earns editing a hotel directory. When the cash runs out, Dr. Isaac tells me he's going to sue my father for unpaid bills if someone doesn't get him to just fill out the fucking insurance forms. I am so scared of my dad's ire that I tell him I hate Dr. Isaac, giving him even less incentive to pay for treatment. I tell my mother that I love Dr. Isaac but that Daddy is trying to turn me against him. I tell each of them whatever it is I think they want to hear because it is the only way to guarantee that either of them will love me. Insofar as a truth existed for me, it changed depending on whether I was with my mom or my dad.

I just wanted two parents who both loved me.

In the midst of all this domestic panic, going away to camp should have been a relief. But it was not. For one thing, the Brendan Byrne Arena was to open that summer at the Meadowlands in New Jersey, and Springsteen would be playing for ten nights as the inaugural act. I got tickets for several of the dates, but the camp director told my mother that I couldn't leave the grounds for anything except a wedding or bar mitzvah, certainly not for Bruce Springsteen. No way.

I told my mother that if that were the case then I simply would not go to camp. No way.

When I called my father and begged him to let me stay at his house for the summer, he mumbled some words about being at work all day and that there was nothing for me to do all alone at home. And I would talk to him about how undisruptive I would be, that I would lie in the sun with iodine and baby oil on and read Dickens and Daphne du Maurier and no one would even know I was there, but he just gave me an emphatic no. He said, It's not possible, and offered no further explanation.

When I hung up the phone, I realized I was really alone in this. Neither of my parents seemed to realize that the end of my tether would be at Seneca Lake, that what little faith I still had would just die and I would go under with it. And it seemed hard to believe that these people who were so close to me couldn't see how desperate I was, or if they could they didn't care enough to do anything about it, or if they cared enough to do anything about it they didn't believe there was anything they could do, not knowing—or not wanting to know—that their belief might have been the thing that made the difference.

I have never felt so lonesome as I did that day when I hung up the phone after speaking to my father, after all he could say was the same old no he always said.

In the end, my Springsteen tickets went to my mother's boyfriend's kids and their friends and I was shipped to camp. But as I got on the bus that summer, instead of telling my mother how much I would miss her, I told her that I was going to get back at her.

Mommy, how can you do this to me? I am so sick and crazy and in such a precarious state of mind and you know it, and I can't believe you're still sending me away like this. How can you do this?

Ellie, you know there's no other choice.

Mommy, if you could only know how far gone I am, you would *find* another choice. You make it sound like I can't do stuff on my own all summer. How bad would it be for me to just hang out and read and see movies? How bad?

You need to be with other kids your age, she said, really hedging. It would be bad for you to stay at home and just get more and more stuck in your own head. Anyway, it's already paid for. Besides, Dr. Isaac said it would be good for you.

Dr. Isaac is a dope. The fact that you've turned him into your guru proves that you're even more of a dope. And I hate you for doing this to me, and as God is my witness I will make you pay.

I did not even kiss her as I approached the stairs to the charter bus. She actually had a camera and was trying to get me to pose with her, arms around each other, while one of the other parents took a shot of us, as if this were all perfectly normal and I wasn't vowing vengeance. I could not figure out why the hell she had to expend so much energy on pretending everything was okay when it so obviously was not. If she put anywhere near as much effort into admitting there was a problem and dealing with it, maybe there wouldn't be one.

As I took my last steps toward the bus, I said to her, If you send me to camp you might as well be sending me to my death.

Oh, Ellie, stop being Sarah Bernhardt, stop being so melodramatic. You'll have fun. Just give it a chance.

I've given it four years. You will live to regret sending me off for a fifth. I swear.

And as I sat on the bus, I thought: All the years. You will pay. I could not think that her life was hard, that she had her own problems, that she needed a break, that there were so many things I wouldn't understand about how difficult it was to be Mommy. I believed then that the pain I was going to feel for the subsequent eight weeks was greater than any justification. No one who had never been depressed like me could imagine that the pain could get so bad that death became a star to hitch up to, a fantasy of peace someday which seemed better than any life with all this noise in my head.

As a child, I remember being left in a lot of different odd places because my mother had to work and my father wasn't there. Weekends and vacations were often spent at my grandparents' house on Long Island, days off from school were spent on organized trips to amusement parks and museums. After a while, in my imagination, summer camp was conflated with the afternoons I spent at Schwartzy's, an after-school place my mother sent me to where all the other kids would play Monopoly or basketball or pinball while I sat in the corner and brooded and read, the only girl in a skirt while all the other children were rugged in their blue jeans and sneakers. The only people I would talk to at Schwartzy's were the women who took care of us, who were always enchanted by my waist-length brown hair and the way I sat still like a little grown-up, legs crossed, posture precise. I couldn't wait until Mommy came to pick me up. The relief of her arrival was so dramatic for me, almost like a wheezing asthmatic who is suddenly given her inhaler: When Mommy arrived, I could breathe freely again.

And here I was, at summer camp, the same kid as ever, stuck in a version of Schwartzy's that lasted eight weeks instead of a mere few hours, lost in a loneliness that felt like forever, like a solitude that would never go away.

On the first day at Camp Seneca Lake, I began a ritual of hanging out in the director's office and telling him that if he didn't throw me out of camp, I was going to take a drug overdose. I explained to Irv that I didn't much want to die, but I knew that I could take enough pills to land me in a hospital, which would mean, at least, that I'd gotten the fuck out of camp. I told him that I'd taken an Atarax overdose a couple of summers before, that everyone had believed it was an accident and I never disabused them of the notion, but now I wanted to make it entirely clear to him that should I take too much of some combination of Motrin and aspirin with maybe a bottle of NyQuil to wash it all down, he could rest assured that I'd acted deliberately, of sane and clear mind and body.

In response, Irv said: You'll ruin your reputation. People talk. Rumors spread. Everyone at all the other camps will find out and everyone you go to school with will find out.

Who did he think he was talking to?

Other days I would tell Irv that rather than hurting myself with pills, perhaps I would just pack a knapsack with some tapes and books and a change of clothes and a tube of Clearasil and walk off the camp grounds one morning and head for the bus station. He told me that the farmers in this most rural and backward area would probably rape me on the road.

After several weeks of our almost daily talks, Irv and I began to develop a strange rapport that could almost be construed as affectionate. Maybe we even begrudgingly liked each other, kind of the way a cop might find himself with a certain distasteful fondness for a murder suspect he is questioning. After hours and hours of listening to anyone's sad luck story in a stuffy interrogation room, it's only natural to start to feel for the poor fool. One day Irv just flat out said to me, in an echo of sentiments I'd heard so many times before, Elizabeth, you're a pretty girl and you're obviously bright enough, so why not just try to be normal? Why not enjoy what there is here at Seneca instead of fighting it so much? There's no reason you can't fit in.

After that remark, it was clear to me that Irv had no idea just how awful it could be to be thirteen. Our negotiations had reached a definite impasse.

I wrote to Dr. Isaac: "I am sitting by the pool and looking up at the clear blue sky. There is an eagle flying across it, and this should be a pretty sight, but it only makes me think of how I long to be free of my human limbs so that I could fly like that bird. I know if I were dead, I would be all spirit and no body, so I pray for my own death." He wrote me back with a bunch of platitudes about how he felt for me in my pain. I responded: "There's no need for you to feel my pain with me. Just get me the hell out of here!"

That summer I was so dogged about wanting out that after a while my plan to take an overdose took on the premeditated tone of a cold-blooded murderer who kills without emotion and later recalls the act with all focus on details and paraphernalia, as if connecting the dots: And then, and then, and then. A perceptible change in my attitude had actually taken place. Because I was so angry at *both* of my parents for keeping me quarantined at camp, I no longer chose sides (some choice, like a criminal on death row who must opt for, say, the electric chair or lethal injection) and my depression turned into a militant rage. Depression has often been described as anger turned inward, so I can see how being infuriated at my parents allowed me the luxury—or perhaps I should say, the salvation—of having that anger at long last turn outward. It was as if I had finally found my strength again in hating the hell out of both of them. And it came as a relief to know that I truly had no one, nowhere, and nothing, that my belief that this whole life thing was just a big sham had been confirmed completely. I could now safely sink into the surrender of what little was left, I could experience the leisure of borrowed time and the pleasure of free-falling. And once I had decided that I was going to commit an act of self-destruction, if that were necessary, I felt released from the harshness of the pain: I had found a way out. Damned if they wouldn't learn themselves a lesson when I left the campground not by bus and not by car, but stretched out in an ambulance and heading for the emergency room.

It was not until some time after visiting day that my father, in what was pretty much his first and last act of paternal authority, came up with a plan of reprieve for me. This gesture of solidarity, of course, didn't involve moving in with him. He had simply arranged for me to stay with his sister Trixie, who lived with her husband and two kids in Matawan, a decaying industrial town in central New Jersey. They had a split-level house with an above-ground swimming pool in the back yard. Bob, Trixie's husband, was a foreman in a factory or something like that, and he was the kind of man who came home and grabbed a Pabst Blue Ribbon at the end of the day and ate his dinner in front of the TV set. The furniture all had plastic coverings, the vegetables came out of a can, ketchup was the main household condiment, Cool Whip and Snack Pak pudding were the basic elements of dessert. In other words, they lived in the blue collar nightmare of my pathetically romanticized Bruce Springsteen dreams. You're finally getting what you want, my mom said when I'd call and describe the setup to her.

Of course, it wasn't really very much fun. In fact, it was absolutely dreary, the kind of experience that made me realize why Springsteen wanted out of this life so badly. All I did all day was hang out, smoke pot, and watch soap operas with my cousin Pamela, who was going to start junior college and major in secretarial science in the fall. But at least I didn't have to go to activities. We went to shopping malls and video game arcades without asking anyone's permission. I went to see Tom Petty at the Capital Theater in August without Irv's blessing. I read whatever abstruse texts I wanted all day and all of the night without anyone interrupting for cleanup or swimming or soccer. I listened to Derek and the Dominos' *Layla*, which had become my album of choice that August. I slept past dinnertime. No one ever questioned anything I did: My father had somehow made it clear to Trixie that I was in a bad way for the moment, and so long as I wasn't bothering anyone else, she ought to just let me be.

Pamela and I seemed to spend a lot of our time driving to Taco Villa or Jack in the Box for lunch, but sometimes I'd go watch her play baseball with her friends, and sometimes she'd take me to one of those late-night back yard keg parties where people do mescaline and peyote and get sick and throw up and slip on each other's vomit and listen to Black Sabbath (which they call just plain Sabbath) and Motley Crue (which they call just plain Crue) and do all sorts of things that sophisticated New York City children would think uncouth. I kind of liked that part of suburbia: I haven't ever been as consistently stoned as I was that summer. Sometimes Pamela and I swam in the pool or sat in the sun—mostly she did the former and I did the latter. Sometimes some of her friends from high school would drop by. All of them were going to community college and majoring in secretarial science, just like Pamela. It was hard for me not to seem like a superior snothead in that environment, so to keep from repelling everyone around me, I tried not to talk too much.

Where on earth would I ever fit in? I kept wondering. At camp everyone is so Jappy, and here in Matawan they're not Jappy enough. Would it be too much to ask to be in an environment where I had *something* in common with the people whose lot I shared? Nothing big: They didn't have to be Springsteen fans. Even Bob Seger or John Cougar would have done the trick. I mean, I was kind of weird as thirteen-year-olds go, but it's not like I needed to be relocated to another planet in order to fit in. Or maybe I did. I was starting to feel that way.

If only I had known the truth about Pamela, if only I'd known we really did have some things in common. It was years later when I found out that Pamela had repeated episodes of depression, of falling into an almost catatonic blankness that made my aunt and uncle so frustrated and clumsy in her presence that they would just scream and prod in their efforts to get her to respond to them. She'd effectively been driven to silence by all the noise, and had an adolescence marked by suicidal behavior. But, of course, we never talked about any of that stuff because who on earth would have thought to bring it up? I didn't know about her, she didn't know about me, and in the cabal of silence and shame that seems so integral to depression, no one had bothered to tell us. So we spent several weeks together bound in this stifled, inarticulate anomie that revolved around *General Hospital* and what was up with Luke and Laura and where to find more weed.

Then, one night on the phone from Trixie's house, my father said, I hope you're not playing your music too loud and driving everyone else crazy. He also said, I hope you're not falling asleep with the TV on like Aunt Trixie tells me you are, because electricity is expensive.

Suddenly, all I could think was that for more than ten fucking years there was this vacuum in my life where a paternal figure should have been, and now he was telling me how to act. It seemed to me that the clock stopped when I was three, and like some latter-day Miss Havisham I was still waiting for my perfect daddy to emerge and rescue me, as cobwebs grew between my molars, as the lacy white cake before me petrified into stone. There was this space filled with nothing but longing for a daddy just like everyone else's. I'd learned to live with this awful sense of lack, and now after all the years he was telling me to behave properly as if he really were my father, and all I could think was, Who the hell is he to tell me what's wrong or right? What the fuck does he know about being a father?

And for the first time, I really understood just how much it must have killed my mother to have him interfere with her parenting. I understood what a violation it is to have someone who has simply not been there all along decide suddenly that he is not just moving in, but taking over. Taking over with words, not with deeds. His love, if I ever cashed it in, couldn't even buy me a morning paper, it was so much about the intangibles that have nothing to do with the workaday requirements of being a parent.

Never in the five summers I had been at camp, not once

in those lonely, homesick days, did I ever want my mommy so badly as I did at that moment.

And I felt so stuck: She was the person closest to me, the only one I trusted, and we were in the most distorted, dependent relationship. I was completely wrapped up in a person who didn't know me at all, like a claustrophobe who chose to live in a small dark cave, trying to whip the fear.

4

Broken

* * *

If you take someone's thoughts and feelings away, bit by bit, consistently, then they have nothing left, except some gritty, gnawing,
shitty little instinct, down there, somewhere, worming round the
gut, but so far down, so hidden, it's impossible to find. Imagine, if
you will, a worldwide conspiracy to deny the existence of the colour
yellow. And whenever you saw yellow, they told you, no, that isn't
yellow, what the fuck's yellow? Eventually, whenever you saw yellow, you would say: that isn't yellow, course it isn't, blue or green
or purple, or. . . . You'd say it, yes it is, it's yellow, and become
increasingly hysterical, and then go quite berserk.

DAVID EDGAR
Mary Barnes

You could think of 1980 as the year that a mandate for con-
servatism and getting the hostages the hell out of Iran got
Ronald Reagan elected president, or as the year John Lennon
was shot to death while signing an autograph as he walked
into his apartment building just off Central Park West. The
slaying took place close enough to where I was lying in bed
at the time that I would later convince myself that I'd heard
the shots, that the random noises of firecrackers, of looting
teenagers and anonymous gunfire all over the place and of
windows and bottles breaking in the projects next door, were
actually specific and purposeful, aimed at rock and roll in
general and John Lennon in particular. For me, it was all just
so much tragedy. It was the year of broken glass and broken
girls, of broken me. It was around that time that my father
walked out for good.

It was then that the noise got to be as loud and frightening as it ever would be, that it went from pathetic to pathological. And it seemed that the only thing that could have possibly stopped the din was the peace, the silence, of my father's withdrawal from the situation, leaving me and my mother alone to muddle through. There was so much bad blood between them, mostly running through me, that one of them had to go, and since my father was the one who lived his life by default, who'd forfeited so much of it to the haze of Valium and the cold comfort of shutting down, it had to be he.

He didn't actually disappear until the end of my freshman year of high school (I was something like fourteen going on fifteen and feeling like I'm a big girl now, who didn't need a father anymore anyway), but the beginning of the end was long before that, maybe as long before as the day my mother first threw him out of the house when I was still a baby.

I remember my graduation from junior high school, the silky purple dress I wore and the Chinese meal of spring rolls and lemon chicken my mother cooked that night, inviting my Grandma and Papa, aunts, uncles, and cousins over to celebrate. My mom made it really clear that she wouldn't allow my dad to come to the ceremony at school, that he couldn't be there to see me receive my diploma because he hadn't helped pay for my education so who was he to suddenly show up now.

I remember trying to explain this to him, trying to tell him why he couldn't attend, telling him something about not wanting to upset Mommy, not being able to come out and say, If you cough up the cash, she'll probably say it's all right, wishing that I didn't have to deal with this. And I remember thinking, I wish one of them would just disappear, never imagining that the worst thing on earth is that sometimes wishes come true.

A lot had changed in the year before he left. He completely stopped paying for Dr. Isaac, and when Mommy ran out of money, my therapy was terminated indefinitely. My mother filed suit against my father because according to their divorce agreement, it was his responsibility to pay my doctor bills. Besides that, his alimony and child support payments had remained at a constant figure since 1969, and she wanted a cost-of-living increase. So they went to court.

Lawyers everywhere. Well, really there were only two, my mother's and my father's, but my dad kept switching firms because no one seemed to think he had a legitimate case. So they multiplied like chicken pox, and every day more and more packets accumulated from the return address of Mr. So and So, Esq., or Benton, Bowl, Beavis, Butthead, and Blah Blah Blah, Attorneys at Law. All of them saying, Elizabeth, there's no need for you to take sides, both of them are your parents, they both love you, and then everyone sneaking up to me and asking, Could you maybe write a letter to the judge about what a lousy father he was? Or else, Do you think you might want to come in and testify? And I'm mostly thinking, Could this possibly be any worse? And I feel a numbness come over me that is, I'm sure, worse than anything ever. It is more like a deep freeze, in which the ice threatens to crack at any moment, but underneath there won't be water, there won't be anything fluid at all, just more and more layers of ice and ice and ice—ice cubes and icebergs and ice floes and ice statues, where a girl used to be.

By then, I was a perfect weirdo by any standard. This was the year of the cheerleader-style miniskirts that Norma Kamali and Betsey Johnson had foisted upon the unfortunately fashion-conscious among us, and all the girls at my high school fell into that category. It seemed that everybody in school was on the cheerleading squad except me, I alone was stuck somewhere in Stevie Nicks-land, showing up every day in these long, diaphanous things that nearly reached the ankles of my leather riding boots, matched with romantic, loosely tied tops that showed off my collarbone. I was all belts and bows and ties and fabric, always weighted down by so much *stuff*, and this was in the beginning of the Reagan-era optimism of the early eighties, the time of lightheartedness and good tidings and bright colors. When all the other girls adorned themselves with plastic earrings and accessories in turquoise and yellow and chartreuse and hot pink, there I was in everything cold and dark, silver and lapis hanging from my ears like an old throwback to the sixties or the seventies, or maybe to an unhappy time and place that everyone who surrounded me didn't remember or had never even been to in the first place.

I tried to fit in a little bit. I even bought a Betsey Johnson velvet party dress with a tight, Lycra bodice and a flouncy little skirt, but I simply felt ridiculous in it, like a circus character who'd accidentally fallen into a Fellini movie when I really belonged in the Nordic desperation of, say, Bergman's *Seventh Seal*. I realized, rather painfully, that the girl I had once been, the one who bossed everyone around, the one who could hold sway over any situation, was simply not coming back. No matter if I ever got out of this depression alive, it made no difference because it had already fundamentally changed me. There had been permanent damage. My morose character would not ever go away because depression was everything about me. It colored every aspect of me so thoroughly, and I became resigned to that.

And in a strange way, this resignation allowed me to stabilize. Sure, I still ran into the girls' bathroom and had crying jags, I still curled into a corner by myself during free periods with the familiar ache, but it had begun to occur to me that all this pain was just a fact of life—or, at any rate, it was a fact of *my* life. I could stay in this state forever. I could do all kinds of things: I could do my homework, I could study for exams, I could write papers and use the standard style for bibliography and endnotes, I could maybe even start dating people who weren't twice my age or half my I.Q. I could actually live the life of a perfectly normal teenage girl—I could, by God, even join the cheerleading squad—but it still wouldn't change that something wasn't right. It still wouldn't change that *I* was all wrong.

I was like a recovered alcoholic who gives up drinking but still longs, daily if not hourly, for just another sip of Glenfiddich or Mogen David or Muscadet; I could be a depressive who wasn't actively depressed, an asymptomatic drone for the cause. But what exactly was the cause? Oh yes, I would remind myself: My goal is getting out of this life, of etching a new identity at some unspecified time in the future when that might be possible. Maybe I could shield myself, refuse to succumb to the symptoms (knowing all too well that one's too many and a thousand ain't enough) just long enough to get out of this rut of a rotten life and get real help, proper help, not Dr. Isaac help, not parental help. I could become the teen machine for a few years, stuck in a zombielike commitment to getting straight A's and appearing absolutely perfect and faultless, on paper.

Instead of thinking that there was *no* future, all I did was plan for the future, treating the present tense and all its tension like a lengthy, labored preamble to a real life that awaited me somewhere, anywhere else but here. I would still be the same girl who spent eight weeks preparing for nothing more than a two-hour ride home from summer camp, only now it would be my adult life that I would be waiting to escape to, believing as I started to believe at the time that if only I could get out of the house and away from the crossfire of my parents' persistent shooting range, maybe I stood a chance.

★   ★   ★

And then Zachary came along, and it wasn't like he was just some guy—he was this astonishingly handsome junior from one of those good families. He was the captain of the tennis team, and by all rights should have been going out with one of those leggy girls in a miniskirt. I know that it is not terribly unusual in the delightful flash of first love to wonder how on earth one has been so blessed, but in my case I was truly baffled. As a couple, we appeared as ridiculously mismatched as Lyle Lovett and Julia Roberts.

Here was this really great, sociable, charming, fun-loving guy who rated so high in all the laundry-list ways that a mother dreams of that he ought to have had GOOD CATCH stamped on his forehead. And he's with, well, me. And everyone's thinking, How can this be? I'd overhear girls talking about us in the school bathroom while I hid in the stall. And I agreed with them completely: If I had been one of those other girls, I'd have made the same catty remarks, I'd have thought that witchy ninth-grader with all that long hair and all those long skirts had nabbed Zachary only because she puts out, or gives good head, or something. To myself, I just thought, Well gosh golly gee, this is my good fortune. With Zachary around, I suddenly felt so shielded, so cosseted and coddled and wrapped up in so many layers of protective coating that everything going down between my parents stopped bothering me. But I kept wondering when the jack-in-the-box was going to pop out and say, Time's up!

My complete absorption in Zachary made it pretty easy not to notice that I no longer saw my father. Dating was such an all-consuming activity: We doubled up with another couple to go to a Police concert (the Go-Go's opened and I sprayed my hair into a bright pink tangle); we went to Zachary's brother's wedding (and of course there was an engagement party before that); we had to blow off school for entire afternoons and go cruising around in Zachary's new

280ZX, as if we were two suburban teenagers; or hide up in his bedroom and make out with the shades closed and the lights off. It seemed that for years I had quietly and surreptitiously prayed to God that He might make me—or whatever it was about me that made me *me*—disappear, metamorphose into somebody else, somebody who didn't walk around as though a crazy, hazy shade of winter hung over even the brightest of days; and after all this time, He sent me Zachary and let me get absorbed into the preternatural ease of life with the perfect boyfriend. At long last, I had disappeared, and this other girl, with this dreamy swain straight out of a Harlequin romance, had taken my place.

And in the midst of this most unlikely spell of wish fulfillment, I refused to let the downs of my dad ruin everything, didn't want to see him and hear about lawsuits or financial difficulties. I didn't want to spend an hour riding back from the few hours a week that we actually spent together, didn't want to do time in the heated car in the middle of winter with him and my stepmother chain-smoking their Winstons, driving along the Throgs Neck Bridge with the windows closed and this horrible sense of suffocation and lung cancer and gloomy, early death all over that Oldsmobile. I was just sick of the whole business of having this unnatural relationship with my father, this strange situation that hadn't changed even years after the divorce. Instead of having ongoing connections with both of my parents, I had to travel between distinct and mutually exclusive universes in order to spend time with either of them. The discontinuity had driven me completely crazy long ago.

And I found myself, so quietly, so subtly, almost completely unconsciously, doing the very thing they told me I never had to do (though they acted like they wished I would): choose between them. And of course, I'm no fool. It was only natural that I side with the person who keeps an apartment with a bedroom in it just for me and doesn't mind when I use whatever soap is by the bathroom sink. We are such extensions of each other, my mother and I, so much two pieces of the same being, that everything that's hers is mine. Of course I chose my mother, for better or for worse.

From time to time I would go through the motions with my father: visiting his mother in her utilitarian housing complex in Brighton Beach, eating Chinese food and revealing to each other what the fortune cookies say. Checking out some new design exhibit at the Cooper-Hewitt, or visiting all the Rembrandts in the Frick Collection. But it wasn't every Saturday. Sometimes it wasn't even every other Saturday. Sometimes it was just once a month, and sometimes it was only a quick dinner in the middle of the week. Sometimes we wouldn't even speak on the phone for a long while. A couple of weeks would go by and we wouldn't even make excuses when we finally hooked up, wouldn't even say, I tried you the other day but there was no answer, because there's no reason to make anything up when everyone understands and tacitly accepts that it's just so much easier this way. It's so much easier not to be torn apart.

Plus, being with Zachary had actually improved my relationship with my mother in ways that five years of five-days-a-week family counseling never could have. My mom liked Zachary so much, she'd practically planned the wedding. She'd make extra-special pasta dishes when she knew I was bringing him home for dinner, and she pretty much decided that, having managed to attract this mensch, I must not be such a mess. She didn't actually say anything to me like, For a few years there it was all pretty much touch and go with you, Ellie. For a few years there I didn't know you would pull through, but now you've got this great guy and everything is just super. She didn't have to say any of this because it was just so obvious, and I didn't have the heart to tell her that it wasn't so, that underneath all that I was feeling as loose and lost as ever.

I want to renounce everything that came before Zachary and deny that there would ever be an after. I start to think, Maybe Zachary and I *will* be together forever and it all really will work out okay. Maybe I *will* marry him. Maybe I *am* Cinderella at the ball. Maybe fourteen isn't too young to know who's right for you, especially since nothing ever seemed right before Zachary. I devote all my energy to thinking about how to keep this relationship from ever ending. I think about it so much that after a while there isn't anything more to the relationship except my plans to keep it going. I mean, for most people, the phone calls, the dates, the schedule that a couple creates, are all a means to an end, a way of organizing time to maximize the pleasure of each other's company. But for me, the time we spend together is about nothing more than furthering that time; every date is about planning the next date, and the next and the next and the next; every phone call is about figuring out when he will call me again, what time, what hour, what minute. Everything is about holding the ideal in place for fear of ever going back to that lonely little world I used to live in.

Then one night, when I am babysitting for our neighbors downstairs, my father calls. Mommy must have told him where he could find me, which I think is a stunning display of maturity on both their parts since they can barely talk without hostility surfacing. I haven't seen my dad or spoken to him in three weeks, and maybe even Mommy is beginning to think this is too long. So we chat. I tell him about Zachary, and for some reason I even tell him that I had gone to Planned Parenthood to get birth control pills.

"I'm glad you're being so responsible," my father says,

ever the laid-back parent, never the moralizer. "Just be care-ful."

"Be careful?" I ask.

"Be careful of your heart."

"Oh that," I say, certain that I have nothing to worry about. "Yeah, well, Zachary's a pretty good guy."

"I know. But be careful."

For the first time in a while, I am taken with sadness that I never see my father anymore. I could never discuss sex with my mother. There are all these things my mother is good for that my father isn't, and all these things my father is good for that my mother isn't, and if only they could work out their differences, or keep the din of discord to a minimum, I could have two whole parents.

"Listen, little one," my father starts to say. "Little one, you know how much I love you."

"Yeah, I guess." I'm not being tentative because I doubt him. I just, I don't know, what the hell can you say when everything's such a mess? What does the word *love* mean in this situation? What good is it?

"Well, Elizabeth, things might happen that you won't understand or that might seem wrong to you, but you should just know that I love you and I'm always thinking about you."

"Okay." I never stop to say, Daddy, what are you talking about? What's going to happen? Because I actually just want to get off the phone so I can call Zachary. My dad had a tendency to speak cryptically and shroud things in mystery when they weren't ultimately that compelling. I kind of thought this was just one of his moments.

I dream that I am a child of two or three, my father is babysitting for me while my mother goes out, and as usual I make him leave his shoes outside my door so I know he's still there. I wake up in the middle of the night, the shoes are gone, but my mother has not come back. I am alone in the house, the electricity is off, I can't get the lights on, I keep bumping into things, I am alone in the dark, I am alone in the world, and I start screaming.

Within a month, my father left New York without a trace, a tragedy that was only eclipsed by the fact that Zachary also left me without a trace, except for the beautiful gold necklace he had bought for me and insisted I keep. He said something about how he wanted to feel like he could play basketball with his friends without worrying that I was going to start crying. And I said that it had never occurred to me that he'd rather be shooting hoops than in bed with me, and he said that, yes, in fact, sometimes he would prefer to play basketball, and that in terms of absolute value, sex and sports were equally meaningless to him, they were just two different ways to have fun.

So all I was to you was a way to have fun? I asked.

Yes. That's right, he said.

And that was it.

Be careful of your heart.

I was, after the breakup, what you call a complete wreck. For the first time in my life, my pain had a focus. And I just couldn't help myself. I didn't care what anyone thought, I didn't care that all the girls in school would say, See, he finally got wise, I didn't care how stupid I would look with teary mascara stains and purple eyeliner tracks down my cheeks, I didn't care about anything except how this was the worst pain ever. I used to weep for never having anything worth losing, but now I was simply resplendent—puffy, red, hysterical—with a loss I could identify completely. I felt justified in my sorrow and I couldn't stand the way everything about Zachary seemed to be everywhere: Every staircase we'd necked on and lounge chair we'd chatted on between classes was redolent with memories of him. My God, even the lint that gathered on my clothing and still hadn't come out in the wash reminded me of Zachary. I would burst into tears in class and not bother to excuse myself. I cried on the subway. One day, I got mugged walking to the subway, and figured it was as good an excuse as any to go home and stay there. Some days, I was so deep in sorrow that every little thing, walking across the street or fixing myself breakfast, was such an effort that I didn't even bother. My hands would go limp as I washed the dishes or applied lipstick. I would fall asleep doing my homework. I would take cabs everywhere because I had no energy to negotiate the public transportation system. My mother felt so bad for me that she would pay for my taxis. I would show up at her office some afternoons and cry. I interrupted business meetings, and if she said she couldn't talk, I would cry some more. My cousin Alison, who was living with us on weekdays at that time, would listen to me review what had happened with Zachary and my plans to win him back. She'd tell me that I was repeating myself and would act amazed when I still went on. My mother and I went on a cruise to Bermuda for Memorial Day weekend, and since there were no phones on the ship, I made them hold the boat in port one day as I gathered enough change to call every one of Zachary's friends at their beach houses to see if he was with them when I couldn't find him at home.

"Elizabeth, you're obsessed and this is crazy! I've had it with this! Had it!" my mother yelled when I returned to our cabin on the ship. "He's not your husband or your fiancé, he's just your boyfriend and there'll be more to come."

There was no way of making her understand that it just wasn't true, that Zachary was my last chance and now it was all over for me.

We're sorry, the number you have dialed is no longer in service. No further information is available.

When my father disappeared, moved far away and didn't tell me where, when I found out because I dialed his number and heard the operator's recording, when my own grandmother wouldn't even tell me where he had gone, when my worst nightmare was realized because my father had at last disappeared, it was almost a relief. My deepest fears had been confirmed, proving that it was not all in my head, that all my years of worrying about everyone disappearing had not been for nought.

I was actually on to something.

As if that could make it hurt any less.

We're sorry, the number you have dialed is no longer in service.

Sorry comes later, years later, with a litany of explanations that shift the blame to circumstances or try to imply that it was all for the best: I left because I hated watching you get caught between me and your mother that way; I left because I was going to start my own business down south, make a lot of money, and be able to take better care of you financially; I left to make life easier for you.

I start to get the weird feeling that nothing is really happening to me, that I am watching a movie and I can turn away any time. I start to think of everything in the third person: A father has walked out on his daughter. *I try to think of odd occurrences and the way one might describe them as if they were someone else's problem:* A husband beats his wife, *I hear an older version of myself saying.* A boyfriend drinks too much and then tries to bash in his girlfriend's face, *I hear another voice from the future reporting. Every personal disaster that might possibly befall me, I can come up with a simple declarative statement to describe.*

The summer after my father leaves, I go on a cross-country trip, and while I'm away, my mother opens my desk drawer, which she knows is my one secret space, but she just wants to throw in a ruler she's found lying around. Her intentions, she swears, were innocent. She doesn't expect to find a foil package printed with the brand name Ortho-Novum, or, sliding the drawer open a couple of more inches, the remainder of my green and white and peach birth control pills.

When I get home from my travels, my mother tells me that she considered suicide when she found the Pill among my belongings. Don't I know that I'm not supposed to have sex unless I'm married? Is it any wonder that things with Zachary turned so bad if we were engaged in this sort of immoral activity? I keep telling her that we never actually had sex, that at some point Zachary and I realized it would be a mistake, but she's not listening.

How can you do this to me? she asks.

To demonstrate how upset she is, my mother opens up my bedroom window and tells me she is going to throw herself out if I don't swear that I'll never do anything like this again. She is raving. She wants me to go to Dr. Isaac for one appointment to talk about why I behave this way.

And she keeps saying, how can you do this to me?

And I want to scream, What do you mean, how can *I* do this to *you?* Aren't we confusing our pronouns here? The question, really, is How could *I* do this to *myself?*

She is hysterical, and it seems crazy to me, just plain wrong, that my boyfriend left me, my father left me, and I am sitting here trying to talk my mother away from the ledge.

What's wrong with this picture? I mean, who died and left *me* in charge?

5

Black Wave

* * *

There's nothing I hate more
 than nothing
Nothing keeps me up at night
I toss and turn over nothing
Nothing could cause a great
 big fight
        EDIE BRICKELL
        "Nothing"

I don't know if I'm running because I'm scared or if I'm scared because I'm running. It's a question I've been asking myself ever since I arrived here at Harvard in September, and I still haven't figured it out. If I stopped for just a minute—stopped speeding from keg party to cocktail party, stopped drinking and drugging, stopped chasing one boy and fleeing from another—if I just said no more *and sat down and did some of my reading for one of my four classes, gave* The Iliad *or* Beyond Good and Evil *a chance, would peace be mine at last? Would the calm I've been waiting for all my life finally get here? Or would it all just be more of so much nothingness like it's always been, like it wasn't supposed to be now that I'm here in enchantmentland, here in this American dream, this university with a name that resonates so far that I sometimes think it could create an echo chamber from here to Australia? I can't believe that even here, even in an institution that seems bigger and better and beyond God the Father, I am still utterly and absolutely just me. Goddamn.*

It wasn't supposed to be this way. I was supposed to be an exotic little American princess, a beautiful and brilliant bespectacled literature student reading Foucault and Faulkner at my rolltop desk in my garret room with hardwood floors, full of whimsical plants and chimes hanging from the ceiling and posters of movie stars from the forties and bands from the sixties on the slightly paint-chipped ivory walls. There were going to be lots of herb tea and a beautiful Mediterranean hookah and paisley cushions and Oriental rugs on the floor so that I could run my own bohemian salon from my guileless little love pad. I wanted a futon with a thick crimson-colored bedspread where I could make love endless nights through sleepy mornings with my boyfriend, a guy who had grown up in Connecticut and played lacrosse and the guitar and me, and who loved me with naughty desire, respect, and abandon.

Where is that girl who all that's happening to? Why is she just so way down?

Why do I spend so much time looking out my dorm room window at Harvard Yard, watching the boys with their jeans slung low on their hips, playing hackysack, kicking little beanbags around on the sides of their Top-Siders like everything is fine, not acting like they're doomed at all? How do I get in on the life happening on the other side of this pane where the world is soft like mud and people aren't afraid to roll in it? What I wouldn't do just to be able to play Frisbee or walk to lecture halls laughing and holding hands, being somebody's baby, being Ali MacGraw in Love Story *or Ali MacGraw in* Goodbye, Columbus, *or anybody else in anything else. My God, where on earth do I have to go to get away from me?*

And I can't stop running. Mostly I am running away from the black wave. It pursues me all over Cambridge. It chases me on those long afternoons when I walk around Harvard Square, roam into one of the zillions of Third World-style stores that crowd Mass. Ave., and maybe try on a pair of long dangling earrings. As I consider the merits of a composition of silver wire and glass beads fashioned into the Himalayan fertility symbols, I take a brief look outside the store-

front window and notice the way the sun is starting to set awfully early, the way it is always so gray and cloudy, the way the dark seems to come so soon and fast and the light never seems to be here at all. And this heaviness falls all over me, even though all I am doing is looking at some earrings in a mirror. I try to concentrate on jewelry, try to think only of bamboo and lapis lazuli, try to imagine this as some kind of Buddhist exercise in deep mindfulness, but I can't because there's this thing creeping up on me, first from behind, then from in front and from the sides and all over, and I feel certain I am being drowned by some kind of black wave. I know that in a moment my feet will be stuck in the wet sand of the undertow, and I must run before it's too late.

I make my way out of the store, I move purposefully back to my dorm room, tracing my footsteps along the cobblestone paths, running from the darkness. I get to the building I live in, fidget with the keys, scurry through the vestibule, hurry up a couple of flights of steps, keep putting the wrong key in the lock, finally get into the suite, finally run into bed, where I hide under the covers and pray that the black wave won't drown me. Pray that if I lie here quietly it will pass. Pray that if I get up in a little while and go to dinner at the Union, that if I just go on with life as if this feeling were normal, the black wave will throw its tidal force at someone else.

But when I unfurl myself from a fetal position and uncurl my way out of bed, there is still an ocean breaking inside my brain. The brief relief of seeing other people when I leave my room turns into a desperate need to be alone, and then being alone turns into a terrible fear that I will have no friends, I will be alone in this world and in my life. I will eventually be so crazy from this black wave, which seems to be taking over my head with increasing frequency, that one day I will just kill myself, not for any great, thoughtful existential reasons, but because I need immediate relief, I need this horrible big muddy to go away right now.

* * *

We drove to Harvard in the rain. My mother and I rode in a white rented station wagon full of my stuff, and full of things I didn't want to bring that she thought I would like, including the shag carpet that used to lie on my bedroom floor when its vivid greens and blues and aquamarines were still fashionable. We were excited as we drove. We stopped at a Howard Johnson's and ate fried clams and pie à la mode and talked excitedly about how exciting it was all going to be. We talked about how I would finally be in "my own element," whatever that meant. We talked about how I would finally be happy.

But the rain was ominous. No denying it. It was the rain that Dylan sings about in "A Hard Rain's A-Gonna Fall." *Where black is the color and none is the number* and all that. I don't like to get too carried away imagining signs from up high, but it rained so hard that I-95 was flooded. There was no visibility, and we had to stop right in the middle of the highway and not move for a while because all the cars had frozen in the dense wetness. And I looked at my mother, and actually said something like, This really doesn't bode well.

And I think she said, Oh, Ellie, don't be silly.

But when we got to Matthews Hall on Saturday afternoon and discovered that I lived on the fifth floor and there were no elevators, even she became a little less optimistic. Even she couldn't figure out how two women were going to get all this stuff upstairs alone, especially in the early September heat and humidity. And she got kind of discouraged and we realized then and there that there was no such thing as salvation without a catch.

When did the running start? Years ago, I'm sure, long before I got to Harvard. I can remember being in high school, walking through Central Park on a chilly day, and the sound of stamping on the crispness of autumn leaves would make me think of the sensation of my head cracking open. And I would get really scared, scared that it would happen and even more frightened that it wouldn't, that a protracted life of misery and wanting to die would go on and on. And I'd run all the way home, running for cover.

But I thought all that was going to stop at Harvard. I thought it was just a matter of getting away from the physical site of so much of my depression. Instead it was even worse; instead the black wave, the gloom, was everywhere. It chased me like a runaway train and clung to me like leeches. And I wasn't just running in a metaphoric sense: I literally didn't stop moving, never dared slow down to think, too scared to find out what was there.

On Halloween of my freshman year, I found myself running through Harvard Yard because my best friend (at least so far), Ruby, was pursuing me and threatening to kill me, her pocketknife unsheathed, screaming something like, You bitch, I'll kill you. She was attacking me because I had stolen her wimpy boyfriend Sam, and she'd just figured it out. The telltale signs: a notebook of mine in his room, a stray earring on his bureau. We'd unexpectedly crossed paths on a precariously narrow staircase that was obviously not big enough for the two of us. But there we both were. I started wishing that the banister was a little bit higher, and a lot more sturdy. Ruby was livid and started to run after me, calling me a whore and a traitor to the feminist cause and a lunatic to boot.

The funny thing is, I didn't really want Sam, Ruby didn't either, and he probably didn't want either of us. She and I had discussed him extensively over the seventeen or so cups of coffee that we tended to down after lunch in the Union, and I knew she had grave misgivings about this effete prepster who read Milton Friedman in his spare time and had arms so weak and thin they could barely even play a decent game of squash, much less hold you and make you feel safe. But I guess in the spirit of the mind games we all seemed to play,

I wanted Sam because he belonged to Ruby, and she wanted him back because he didn't want her any longer. I understand now that if we'd all just done our homework and gone to bed before midnight and woke up in time for morning classes—if we'd lived like normal people—all this nonsense could have been completely avoided. We'd have been too busy in the purposeful pursuit of life to participate in this kind of sideshow. But we weren't. We were all nuts and desperate. We couldn't help creating this love-triangle psychodrama out of the nothingness that drove all three of us, all of us being completely crazy, sad, empty.

You see, it was no longer just me. Harvard was full of nut cases, and we'd all managed to find each other, as if by centrifugal force. Still, no one's desperation came close to matching mine. People at school were sufficiently eccentric to offer a new playground for my neuroses, to create novel opportunities for acting out. But in the end, after the curtain dropped over these little dramas, they all seemed able to go back to their rooms and back to their lives, they all seemed to know that it was just a game, that it scuffed you up and wore you out a little, but that you would get on with it. Only I seemed to be left behind, crying and screaming about wanting more, wanting my money back, wanting some satisfaction, wanting to feel something. I was the only person going to a prostitute in search of true love. But somehow, no matter how often I was disappointed, I was always game for the next round, like a drug addict hoping that a new fix will give him a rush as good as the first one. Only I'd never even had the initial euphoria that makes a junkie keep coming back for more. I always sought solace in places where I knew, absolutely, that it did not exist.

And I knew, as Ruby chased me just beyond the Yard, toward the Science Center, that I had finally crossed some line. It all became so clear to me. I knew that *this was insanity*:

Insanity is knowing that what you're doing is completely idiotic, but still, somehow, you just can't stop it.

I was scared of the way I felt as I ran away, knowing that
if I stopped, I might have to confront the reason why I was
always running—and I'd have to admit that there was no
reason. Run, run, run. Was it toward something or away from
something else? The senselessness of this display was too upsetting to contemplate. Just as all my previous machinations
for escaping from the demons in my head had failed, this latest
scheme wasn't going to work out either. Sam wasn't just a
boy to me. He was yet another version of salvation. His father
was the president of a major motion picture studio, and when
Sam approached me in the cafeteria and said he was going to
take me to Los Angeles and take me out of my life and out
of my mind, when he said we could write screenplays, when
he said, Hey, baby, I'll make you a star—when he said all
these things, I knew they were lines, and still I bought them.
He said we could go to his house in the Bahamas for winter
break. He said we could go to Cannes for the festival. He
said, he said, he said. And I believed him. I imagined a buf-
fered universe of sunshine and safety. I dreamed of going off
to a never-never land where scary moods and ugly thoughts
and black waves just didn't exist. For a few days, while planning my transport, via Sam, to a place where nothing bad
ever happens, I was almost in decent spirits. I could concentrate on reading Hegel for more than a minute at a time.

I could not bear the thought that I was going to be de-
nied this escape fantasy because Ruby had convinced Sam to
come back to her. I could not bear the deep freeze settling in
around my bones at the thought that yet another attempt to
get out of my life alive would end in disappointment. Time
became palpable and viscous. Every minute, every second,
every nanosecond, wrapped around my spine so that my
nerves tightened and ached. I faded into abstraction. A self-

generated narcosis created a painful blank where my mind used to be. It was only when Ruby saw the look on my face that she stopped yelling, saw that I was more of a threat to myself than to her or anyone else's happiness.

She said, What's wrong with you? Say something! Tell me how you can do this to me!

And all I could say, to no one in particular, was, Please don't leave me, don't leave me here to die, don't leave, don't go.

What's wrong with you, Elizabeth? Why don't you talk to me? Why don't you say something? Why don't you defend yourself?

I wanted to say, I can't, I've receded, I'm lost. I wanted to say so much but I just couldn't.

You're crazy, Ruby said. You should seek counseling.

And I wanted to say to her, You know, you're right.

Instead I walked away from Ruby lost in vertigo. The Yard seemed like a phantom. I moved through it in the plastic bubble that separated my fogworld from everything around me. It was dark and gray, and dead leaves crunched under my penny loafers, reminding me of that old sensation of my head cracking open. I passed friends who said hello. But I could barely see or hear them. Their voices seemed to be coming from somewhere else, like a movie whose soundtrack was not in sync with the visuals. Or maybe it was more like home movies, everything flashing by me in clipped, grainy frames, with the click-click-click of the projector buzzing in my ears. So I just kept walking quick and straight, an automaton following a program.

I walk toward the University Health Services building. Through the glass doors. Through revolving doors inside. Still breathing. In one door of the elevator. Out the other door at the third floor. Follow the arrows to MENTAL HEALTH. *Into the west wing. Ask to see a*

psychiatrist. The receptionist says that only a psychologist is available.
Minutes later, walk into Dr. King's office. Tell him I need help.
Really badly. Tell him I am scared. Tell him that it feels as if the
floor beneath my feet is crumbling, that the ceiling is about to land
on my head. Tell him I feel like an art deco skyscraper, like the
Chrysler Building, but my foundation is crumbling and shattered
glass is falling all over the sidewalks, all over my feet. I am walking
barefoot on broken glass in a very dark night. I am collapsing and I
am collapsing on myself. I am shards of glass, and I am the person
being wounded by the glass. I am killing myself. I am remembering
when my father disappeared. I am remembering when Zachary and
I broke up in ninth grade. I am remembering being a little child and
crying when my mother left me at nursery school. I am crying so hard,
gasping for breath, I am incoherent and know it.

Dr. King checked me into Stillman Infirmary for a couple of
days, where they let me rest, where they let me chill out for
a little while so that I would be able to go back out into
Harvard Yard and do all the same stupid things all over again.
Well, actually, that's not what they thought. They thought
that this break from activity would give me perspective. But
sadly, I knew better: This break is nothing but time-out, take
five, recess. Lying in bed for a few days wouldn't help enact
the kind of personality overhaul it would take to pull me away
from my well-established pattern of mapping out escape
routes, clinging to them like vines, and then watching as these
lifeless forces suddenly pushed me away, though I continued
to hold on for dear life. I knew I would find another Sam, I
knew I would find another way to pretend, even just for a
little while, that I didn't feel so lousy. I always did. In the
meantime, the people at Stillman fortified me for my next
round of mishaps, feeding me simple meals of boiled chicken
on Styrofoam plates, bringing me Dalmane at bedtime to be
certain that I got plenty of sleep. When they were satisfied

that I wasn't going to do myself in, they let me leave, but insisted that I must be in therapy, I couldn't be trusted without it. And I didn't know how to tell them the extent of my insurance problems, and how much trouble I had talking about money with my parents, and that the hassle it would take to get someone to pay for therapy might do more damage than just trying to get on with life. Amazingly, Dr. King agreed to call my father and make arrangements, so that my bills would be paid through IBM's employee benefits office without my involvement.

It is the nicest thing, I think, that anyone has ever done for me.

If boys weren't confusing enough, drugs addled the situation even more. Ecstasy had not yet been scheduled by the D.E.A. in any of the agency's illicit categories, so the little white capsules that looked like a vitamin supplement and felt like a nitroglycerin love bomb going off in your cerebral cortex were still perfectly legal during my freshman year. I didn't like pot, I didn't like cocaine, I didn't like drinking (though I seemed to do all of them anyway), but Ecstasy was sweet relief for me. On an Ecs trip, I got to be away from myself for a little while. It was never long enough, I always wanted more, always wished the drug had a longer half-life than it did, but for a little while, when I was rushing on that Ecstatic run, all was quiet on the western front of my mind.

Until it got out of hand. We started to do so much of it so often that around campus people began to refer to Ruby, our other pal Jordana, and me as the Ecstasy Goddesses. At parties, we walked up to people who we didn't know and told them how much we loved them. On Ecstasy, we were best friends with everybody, we no longer felt the class distinctions that were all over Harvard, we no longer felt poor and ugly. We could escape the wide gulf of circumstance that separated the three of us, with our overworked, overtired single mothers, with our scholarships and student loans, from the boys we seemed to keep hooking up with, the ones with last names like Cabot and Lowell and Greenough and Nobles. All of them seemed to have gone to Andover and Hotchkiss and were at Harvard as legacies, as "development cases" (the code phrase the admissions office uses for the children of major money donors), all of them substandard students who the school insisted take a year off before entering. Why all of us, we smart urban Jewish girls who worked as waitresses and typists to earn tuition money, chose to take up with these guys for whom Cliffs Notes were invented is beyond me. But we did. It was pretty obvious that they hung with us because they wanted a break from all the blondes who played field hockey, the girls they'd known forever from summers in Maine or NOLS courses or prep school. But why we allowed ourselves to be swayed by their money and their cocaine is still a mystery. Maybe I thought it was part of the Harvard experience. Maybe I thought it was what I was supposed to do. Maybe it seemed the only logical conclusion to the disappointment of Harvard: I'd spent all my time in high school getting good grades, editing the newspaper and literary magazine, taking dance classes, doing whatever else, all because I wanted to go to a great college like Harvard and be transmogrified. But once I actually got there, once I discovered that the air in Cambridge didn't tingle, once I found out it was a place like any other only more so, once I realized that my classmates were not glamorous sophisticates but just a bunch of hormones on legs like teenagers throughout the country, I think I decided I might as well drug my way through. *Pass the pills and fancy plants / Give us this day our daily trance.* Whatever the reason, somehow I found myself, the girl who was scared of drugs because a mind is a terrible thing to waste, wanting to be wasted all the time.

Three days before winter break, I realize I have bottomed out when I wake up in Noah Biddle's room on a Sunday morning after an Ecstasy trip the night before. Noah is the heir to a banking fortune, an Andover boy from Philadelphia's Main Line who is such a brat that when Harvard told him he had to take time off before entering as a freshman, he actually hired a consultant to plan the year for him. He does so much coke that I have started to wonder how he will look with a third nostril. I don't really like him much, but for some reason I will do anything to get him to like me, an impossible task, because he just doesn't. I keep thinking that if I could only win Noah's love, I would finally feel as if I've actually arrived at Harvard, appended myself to someone so integral to the place, so at home here, so at home on this earth and in his own skin in a way that I will never be, that the minefields in my head would stop exploding at long last.

So here I am, lying nearly naked on the carpet in the common room of his suite, my head pillowed by a puddle of beer. Noah is next to me on the floor, we are wrapped in each other the way dried, harried flowers stick together after a week in a vase. In my parched exhaustion, I can just barely survey the debris of last night's mess: Since everyone smokes and chews gum with Ecstasy, there are ashes and little sticky pink blobs attached to the coffee table and the floor; because everyone feels so agile on Ecstasy when in fact they are extremely clumsy, there are spilled bottles and empty plastic cups. There are items of clothing everywhere, mostly mine. But I can't see a clock through the blur of my desiccated contact lenses that I should have taken out hours before, and I need to know what time it is because my grandparents are supposed to visit and I've got to meet them at my room sometime before noon. When I finally can see my watch, can see that it's past 4:00 P.M., that they have probably already come and gone, and that besides I've got a paper due tomorrow that I haven't even thought about yet, I feel a panic come over me that doesn't quite erupt because the residual effect of the Ecstasy preempts it. But somewhere deep down inside under all the anesthesia, I know I have really fucked up big time. I know that nothing is as it should be, nothing is even the way I wish it would be. I've slept through my grandparents' visit, I might as well sleep through the rest of my life, and I am so horrified that I let out the loudest scream I've ever made.

Noah pops up, frightened of how frightened I am, tries to silence me, says people will think I'm being raped or murdered, but I can't stop screaming. I try, but I just can't. He's petrified, he's wishing he never got mixed up with me, he's looking at me like I'm a tornado or a dust storm that's just outside his window, way beyond his control, and he's praying that the damage will be minimal. I keep screaming. Being a veteran preppy stoner, Noah is so used to acid freak-outs in the middle of Grateful Dead shows that he knows how to cope, knows how to get into an adrenaline-induced dealing mode. He puts on his clothes, manages to get me into mine, covers my mouth with his hand as he picks me up and walks me out the door and into the emergency room at University Health Services, me screaming all the way, all the way through the Yard and the snow and the freezing cold.

Noah leaves me there, leaves me with a nurse who shuffles me into an examining room. I am sure I will never see Noah again. I start to think that never seeing him again is even worse than how bad I feel about my grandparents. The nurse calls the psychiatrist on duty. She won't let me leave even though I keep saying, I've got to see my grandparents, they're waiting for me, we have to get brunch, they're eighty years old, they drove up here from New York this morning.

The nurse explains that it's too late anyway, that it's five in the evening. But I just keep saying, I've got to find my grandparents. I might as well be Dorothy, clicking the heels of my ruby red slippers together, repeating the words *There's no place like home.* If only we were in Oz.

They ask me if I've done any drugs in the last twenty-four hours, and I say no. Then I say, I guess I smoked some pot and snorted some coke also, but that was just to make the Ecstasy last longer. I also admit to them that I had some beer, maybe a couple of sea breezes somewhere in there, too. And then the doctor asks if I have a substance abuse problem, and all I can do is laugh. I laugh really hard and really loud, a howling hyena laugh because what I'm thinking is how nice it would be if my problem were drugs, if my problem weren't my whole damn life and how little relief from it the drugs provide. I keep laughing, on and on, like a nut, until the doctor agrees to give me some Valium and keeps me, half prone, on the adjustable examining table until I calm down. Maybe an hour goes by. In its quiet, gentle way, the Valium flattens my hysteria into a mere lack of affect, and after many assurances that I will be just fine, really I will, the doctor sends me on my way, telling me to get some rest over winter vacation.

When I get back to my room, there are eight messages from my grandparents, calling from various points in Cambridge, the final one saying that they're going home. My hallmates, who say they tried to call me all morning at Noah's but there was no answer, look at me like I'm a really bad person. They look at me like I'm the kind of person who would sleep through her octogenarian grandparents' visit after they have driven five hundred miles in one day just to see her—and of course, that's exactly the kind of person I am. Brittany says, *Maybe you should take some time off.* Jennifer says, *What's wrong with you? Everyone goes crazy sometimes, but how can you do this to your grandparents, they're these little people, they were so worried?* And all I can do is go into my room and crawl into bed.

When I wake up, after a Valium sleep that makes me think I'm turning into a creep like my dad, I call my political philosophy section leader (it seems fitting that the course is called Justice) and tell him that I can't hand my essay in tomorrow because I slipped on some ice and got a concussion. The girl who never once submitted a paper a day late, the girl who lived for the small amount of structure that deadlines provide for a mental state running rampant, seems to have decided that all that good stuff doesn't matter anymore. That girl is gone. She is going home for winter break and never coming back.

The thing is, there was never any pleasure, no element of partying in any of the drug use and abuse I was involved with. It was all so pathetic, so sad, so psychotic. I was loading myself with whatever available medication I could find, doing whatever I could to get my head to shut off for a while. Maybe for Noah, who was pretty much a happy-go-lucky child of a happy home, coke and Ecstasy were all about being party-hardy (I can remember his silly delight as he taught me how to do a bong hit, how to snort a line of cocaine without blowing it off the mirror like Woody Allen does in *Annie Hall*), but for me it was all desperation. It wasn't just recreational drug use. I would find myself, whenever I was in anyone's home, going through the medicine cabinets, stealing whatever Xanax or Ativan I could find, hoping to score the prescription narcotics like Percodan and codeine, usually prescribed following wisdom tooth extraction or some other form of surgery. On Percodan, which is nothing less than an industrial-strength painkiller, I almost felt no pain. I would hoard those little tablets, save them up for a big pain emergency, and take them until nothing much mattered anymore.

But I never had enough money or adequate street smarts to actively pursue any kind of drug habit. I relied on happenstance, on other people's provisions, for whatever drugs I was taking. But it was mostly to no avail: Whatever relief a brief drug trip gave me was never enough. And I was not a very good user: I often had the kind of freak-outs that led me to the emergency room and left everyone else I was hanging out with swearing that they'd never get fucked up with me again, I wasn't worth the trouble I often caused. Only two days after Noah took me to U.H.S. for my post-Ecstasy panic attack, I was back at the E.R. in the middle of the night looking for some Thorazine because I'd smoked so much pot that I became convinced that my foot had a life of its own, kind of like one of those people with multiple personality disorder whose hand writes things that her head doesn't know about. And then I thought the walls were closing in on me, and when I lay in my bed I was certain the sword of Damocles was hanging over me, and I was sure that if I went to sleep I would wake up dead.

Basically, drugs were no solution to any of my problems. I was a klutz with a joint in my hand, so inept at chemical self-destruction that I often was reminded of the story about Spinoza trying to kill himself by drowning, but failing because his foot got stuck in the dock. My God, how much I wanted to be sane and calm on my own! I would have loved nothing better than to see my grandparents, to take them around Cambridge, to show them Harvard Yard, Widener Library, the entryway to Adams House with the beautiful gold-flecked mosaic ceiling. I would have loved to take them to Pamplona or Algiers or Paradiso or one of the other cafés where I would spend long, lazy hours reading and gossiping and drinking double espressos to stay awake. I would have loved to show them that I was all right after all, that their lonesome little grandchild who always seemed so bookish and morose had really turned out okay.

During my senior year of high school, my first cousin (one of their other grandchildren) had married a Wall Street tycoon, had celebrated with a huge wedding at Windows on the World, and had made the whole family so damn proud by making such a good match. I knew I would never do anything like that, I knew I was attracted mostly to hopeless hippies and other lost souls like me, but I wanted my grand-parents to be impressed with the things I could do: I could write, I could study, I could get into Harvard. I looked for-ward to their visit with about the same amount of glee that a former fat girl who has slimmed into a glamorous woman looks forward to her tenth-year high school reunion. Noah could have come to brunch with us—at least, in my fantasy he would have—and even though he wasn't Jewish, he was a charming Pennsylvania Yankee, his sisters had made their society debuts all over the Northeast, and my grandparents would have headed back home to Long Island thinking of me as a stunning collegiate success.

Instead, they were just worried, scared stiff, wondering what the hell had happened to their youngest grandchild, the one who used to come to their house every weekend and on every vacation when she was little because her mother worked and her father slept and there was no one to take care of her. They had practically raised me, and now they would wonder what had gone wrong. There was no way I could possibly explain to them that I was suffering from an acute depression, that it was so intense that even when I wanted to get out of my own head and attend to other people's needs—as I had so much wanted to do that day—I just couldn't. I was consumed by depression, and by the drugs I took to combat it, so that there was nothing left of me, no remainder of the self that could please them even for a few hours. I was useless.

Winter break, all I do is hide in my room at home. I think I might actually be going through some kind of withdrawal. The semester has been too tumultuous. I know it's normal to endure some kind of adjustment period when you first go off to school, but this sure doesn't feel normal to me. I can't even pretend that everybody else has the same problems that I've had because I'm still the only person I know whose best friend chased her through Harvard Yard with a knife, and I'm still the only person I know (though I'm sure there must be others) who moved from a suite in Matthews Hall to a single in Hurlbut, citing mental instability as the main reason that I could not bear to live with other people. It's true, fair enough, that everyone at school has troubles aplenty, but they all seem to have settled into their situations and forged whatever imperfect form of peace, whatever entente of convenience, makes life bearable. But not me. Oh no. I will always be a runner. I will always be looking over my shoulder, or, if someone is trying to talk to me, over *his* shoulder, at the next available opportunity, the next brass ring I might grab onto. It is only now, here at home, that I can come to a safe stop.

One night my mother walks into the apartment after work and comes into the dark recesses of my room, where I have been lying, in the same red flannel nightshirt, since the day I got back from school. I have mostly been doing my reading for Justice class, amazed by how engrossing it can be, how much I can learn from Kant's *Grounding for the Metaphysics of Morals* or Mill's *On Liberty* or John Rawls's *A Theory of Justice*. Maybe if I had just spent more time with my books, first semester would have been less destabilizing. Maybe if I can keep reminding myself that Harvard is, contrary to common myth, just a school—and not, say, some group home for misguided youth—I might actually get something worthwhile out of the place. Hadn't I always retreated to the splendid isolation of my studies?

My mother sits down on the spare bed in my room, still wrapped in her insular fur-lined coat as if the chill from outside were in here too. She starts turning on lights, flicking the switch for the overhead lamp, the darkness of winter at 6:00 P.M. is too much for her, and I don't know if she'll understand that the little reading lamp that I have been using gives about as much brightness as I can stand right now. I don't know if she sees that I am in hiding.

"This place is filthy," she says. "Elizabeth, you're either going to have to clean up in here or leave the house. I can't live with this mess."

Well, I can't move, I want to say, but don't. "Mom, can't you see I'm too depressed to do much of anything, including cleaning? Anyway, it's my room. What's it to you if it's messy?"

"It's my house, and I will not live this way!"

She starts fussing with her hair, pulling at the curls and twirling them on her fingers. She can't stand to see me this way, can't quite come to terms with the fact that the mess of my room is the least of it.

"Listen, Elizabeth, your term bill from Harvard for next semester just arrived, and even with your grants and loans, it's still a lot of money."

"I know."

"Do you? Do you really know? Because I've always paid the bills for you, always made sure you had what you needed even if I didn't have enough for myself, so I'm sure you don't know the value of money. It's my own fault for spoiling you

the way I did." She shakes her head, and I can see she's starting to cry, and I think, Oh no. "If you knew the value of
money I'm sure you wouldn't be wasting your education
away like you are, partying and doing whatever else it is you
do," she continues, all tears. I begin to interrupt her, to say
something about how it isn't as fun as it looks, that higher
education ain't what it's cracked up to be, but she waves her
hand at me to shut up. "Look, I don't know what it is you
do up there and I have a feeling I don't want to know. But
it makes me sick that you're just having a good time while I
slave away every day, while I work so hard and have to count
every penny so that you can go to Harvard. And now I see
that I send you off there, and you come back a complete mess,
and I want to know what's going on! I want to know, or else
I won't pay your term bill."

"You just said you didn't want to know."

"I don't." She starts to really cry. "It's just that I feel like
I worked so hard to raise you well, and I did it all by myself,
I never had anyone else to turn to, and I've tried so hard to
be a good mother, and then you go off to Harvard and it
seems like all the good things I brought you up to believe
don't matter anymore. You don't care whether the boys you
date are Jewish and—" She starts to wail, her face contorting
strangely like she's about to have a seizure. "And you do all
these . . . all these . . . all these—"

"All these what? What, Mom?" I run over to hold her
so she will stop crying. Whatever problems I have, hers always
seem worse.

"All these drugs." She gasps. "Oh God, Ellie, I can't
take it. Not my baby. I can't watch this happen to you.
I've been so upset. You're going to send me to an early
grave."

"Mom, what gives you the idea I'm doing drugs?"

"Because if you weren't on drugs, you wouldn't have

missed your grandparents when they came to visit you. You're selfish as can be, and the only person you ever think about is you, but even you, even you wouldn't have just let your grandparents drive all the way up there to see you and just not be there." More bawling.

"But, Mom, I already told you that I was in the infirmary because I fell over the night before and had a concussion."

Did anyone really buy this?

"You just fell? Is that what you're telling me? You expect me to believe that?!"

I guess not.

"I slipped on ice. It's cold in Cambridge, much colder than New York."

"Oh, Elizabeth. Stop lying. Even if you did fall it was because you were on drugs." She pauses to catch her breath, and her face looks quizzical and obtuse, like she's trying to work on one of those long calculus problems that are so labyrinthine that by the time you find a way to figure it out, you can't even remember the question. "Actually, I have no idea what's going on up there. Probably it isn't drugs. I have no idea. No idea."

I'm relieved that she's moving away from the dope hypothesis because there's no way I'll ever be able to explain it to her. Still, she's not abandoning it altogether. "Just look at you," she says. "You look horrible. Everyone else goes away to college and gains weight, but you're skinnier than ever and it's probably from drugs. I even see you here at home. You barely eat."

She has a point about my weight. I left for school at five five and at least 120 pounds; when I weighed myself just a week ago I was down to about 100, light enough, I reminded myself, to be in Balanchine's corps de ballet, where all the girls had to be skinny and swanlike, where so many of the girls were crazy from drugs and starvation. I never wanted to be crazy like a dancer. I never wanted to be crazy like me.

"Maybe I'm just depressed," I suggest to her, hoping that the truth might set us free of this miserable conversation. "Why blame external things like drugs? You always say, It's Daddy's fault for leaving you, or It's because you grew up in the City. Now you're saying I'm such a mess because of Harvard. Why don't you consider the idea that I might just be, at the core, completely depressed? Maybe it's just the way I am. Maybe I was born under a bad sign. Maybe I really do need drugs to make me feel better, the kind that doctors prescribe."

"Maybe." She sighs. I know what she's thinking: Why is this never easy? She's calmed down a bit, the loud, hysterical crying has mellowed into a resigned whimper. "The doctors always said there was nothing wrong with you chemically, that it was emotional. They said they could fix you." Then the wailing starts again. "Look, Elizabeth, I know everyone goes through some trouble, but not everyone steals friends' boyfriends or moves out of their original room or parties all the time like you do. And nobody completely misses her grandparents when they come to visit." She is screaming tears. "What were you thinking that day? They're old people, they're over eighty. They don't know what's going on. They don't understand where you were. They're simple people, and maybe they're not perfect, and maybe you wish you had other people for grandparents, maybe you wish you had a family more like you, but they love you. They really love you. What's wrong with you? Tell me!"

What can I say? I am rotten, so rotten that I wish I were anyone but me. I wish I were dead. I try to think of some explanation for my depression that will make sense to her, but I can't imagine what will. I can't even explain it to myself. I can't even look her in the eye, and say, Well, I had a tough childhood, because it sounds like a line, an excuse, a boulder I've conveniently placed on my shoulder so that I can live with all my misery. It's not like I was beaten regularly, it's not like I was raised by wolves, it's not like I'm an exceptional case: I am just one of a whole generation of children of divorce whose parents didn't handle their personal affairs very well and who grew up damaged. Could family dynamics possibly account for all this trouble? Was my brain chemistry part of the problem too? Who the hell knows why I'd gone so far wrong, but the plain fact was that I had. I couldn't get out of bed, I couldn't eat, I couldn't change into different clothes, I couldn't even explain myself to my mother.

"Mommy," I say, and I start to cry in spite of myself. "Mommy, you don't know how hard it was for me to know how hard it was for you. I hated being the only child, I hated being so dependent on you because Daddy was out of it, and I hated the way you were so dependent on me. I never got to be a little kid. I never got to just have fun. And you never got to just enjoy motherhood. It was always so much pressure. You were always trying to please me, and I was always trying to please you. I always wanted to be better than everyone else in your family, better than all my cousins my age because I always felt like I wasn't good enough to them because I didn't have a father like everyone else." More crying on my part and hers. "But, see, I was good enough. I really was. I was the best little girl in the whole wide world to begin with. Don't you remember that? Don't you remember me? You see, I remember me, even if no one else can. I remember trying so hard, and I remember that *no one ever told me I was good enough!* All I ever wanted to do was be a happy kid, but I was always this little adult, and no one ever told me *I was a good kid!*"

I am starting to ramble, and I am embarrassed to see that I have overshot my goal: I wanted to say something that could illuminate the nature of my sorrow for my mother's benefit, but instead I am getting taken in by the pathos myself. What I am saying sounds like a speech in one of those movies that might star Tom Cruise, a film that explores any of a roster of major tragedies—the Cultural Revolution in China, the Vietnam War, the Holocaust, an I.R.A. bombing in London—and still in the face of all this genuine, world-rocking sorrow, all of the protagonist's troubles will be portrayed as nothing more than a lack of self-esteem. Films like this suggest that international disasters can be caused or curtailed by mothers who love too much or not enough, by fathers who disappear, or appear only as abusive alcoholics. I am all too aware that as I sit talking to my mother, I am beginning to sound like a Hollywood cliché, and yet I know that a lot of stock characters are built on some real truths. I know that sometimes the personal is political, that people who could make the world a better place end up adding to its destruction because they are fucked up, they're from bad homes. So I just continue with my babbling.

"I thought getting into Harvard would prove to you and everyone else that I was good enough," I say. "I thought if I could get into Harvard, everyone would finally say she's okay, she's a good kid. But now you're yelling at me, and soon your sister will probably call and yell at me because of what I did to Grandma and Papa, and your whole family is going to say that I'm an awful kid, but in the meantime I'm trying so hard. I'm trying so hard. Trying so hard. Trying . . ."

By now, my mother is hysterical, I'm hysterical, we are wrapped in each other's arms, my mother still in her heavy coat, me still in this flannel nightshirt that is like a second skin. "All I ever wanted was for you and everybody to love me just the way I am," I whisper into her fur collar, not caring if she doesn't hear, I don't know why I'm talking anymore anyway. "But now I just hate everybody. I don't care about anyone else because I'm so hateful."

"Oh, Ellie, I know," my mother says. "I know. And I'm so sorry."

6

Happy Pills

✳ ✳ ✳

People like us, who believe in physics, know that the
distinction between past, present, and future is only a
stubbornly persistent illusion.

ALBERT EINSTEIN

Harvard, in its infinite wisdom, followed two weeks of vacation with one week of reading time and three weeks of
finals, which meant that there was no reason to do any work
at all during the semester proper. All of it could be saved for
those six accumulated weeks of rope from which to hang
what was left of your mind after all that nothing, all those
meandering Cambridge days that were occasionally interrupted by classes. Of course, after a vacation that amounted
to my own version of house arrest, I was back in school, same
as ever. Even in my lowest moments of lolling about my
bedroom, I knew that in the end I'd return to school, take
finals, get good grades, and get through second semester. At
heart, I have always been a coper, I've mostly been able to
walk around with my wounds safely hidden, and I've always
stored up my deep depressive episodes for the weeks off when
there was time to have an abbreviated version of a complete
breakdown. But in the end, I'd be able to get up and on with

it, could always do what little must be done to scratch by.

One night during my first exam period at Harvard, after dinner I was sitting in my room trying very hard to concentrate on *The Odyssey* and having no luck. I know it was supposed to be a fun read, a trippy epic full of Sirens and Lotus-Eaters, island romance with Calypso, and poor Penelope weaving and unraveling at her loom, warding off her suitors, waiting, waiting, waiting, the avatar of feminine virtue, for her dear, wayward Odysseus to come back home. *The Odyssey* was one of those books that people loved, thought was way better than *The Iliad*, which was all just soldiers and battlefields and macho jockeying for position, but I just couldn't muster up the slightest bit of interest in all the ancient globetrotting. My thoughts kept roaming elsewhere. It was amazing to me the way I could go home and peacefully read for a couple of weeks—even manage to escape from the moody blues and ugly blacks through the deep concentration of books—but now, back at school, I got shaky again. My whole body would vibrate, my head would start to hurt, and my mind would wander to the world outside my room where I was sure that all my friends were having a good time and feeling completely relieved not to have me around to deal with.

And it wasn't just because every time I got stoned I ended up in the emergency room, usually dragging a helpless, addled entourage along with me. Even when I was okay, I was still a nuisance: My presence created a tension that would disturb the mellow vibe that was central to preppy party rituals. It was never enough for me just to go to a party and enjoy the company, it was never enough to play quarters or other dumb drinking games. There had to be more, some point, some grandiloquent promise of redemption, and it didn't matter who I bopped on the head in the process of trying to find it. It seems my behavior was so disruptive that finally Noah had to say that he loved me dearly, really he did, but I could hang out in his room only if I promised to sit quietly and listen to music and not do drugs. But Noah's room was nothing less than an opium den. There was no reason to be there sober.

So I tried staying in my room and reading like I was supposed to. But I couldn't make it through another page. The missing-father theme in *The Odyssey* must have had some subliminal effect on me because I picked up the receiver and dialed my dad's number in Florida. He'd settled into a cute little white hacienda house, the kind with tiled floors and throw rugs and wicker furniture and pillows in shades of peach and seafoam, and a kidney-shaped pool in the back yard that overlooked the Intracoastal. Life had not been bad for him since he'd gone away. In fact, it was impossible not to notice that life had been a lot better in the four years since he'd cleared his daily docket of any dealings with me and my mom. I resented the hell out of him for his ease, his luxury, his ability to live out the dream we all have that if we ignore our annoyances, they will go away. Despite his attempts to tell me at various points over the years after he'd left that there was a piece of his mind that was consumed with thoughts of me, that there was a part of me that never left his conscious life, I didn't believe him. I was so much easier for him to forget.

Ever since my father had left, he and I had these twice-a-year reconciliations, kind of the way department stores have semiannual sales: Crowds flock to them expectantly, only to find that what remains once they arrive is all just junk anyway. We'd get together with the best of intentions, I'd keep swearing to myself that I'd forgive him for abandoning me, while he'd promise himself that he wouldn't let his guilt overwhelm him. We'd have a few pleasant conversations, and then I wouldn't hear from him for another six months. And then we'd go through all the emotional trauma of *you're a terrible father / your mother made it impossible for me to stay* all over again.

A whole year had passed since my father's move to Florida before he called me. He had come up to New York for some reason, had run into my mother in, of all places, Bloomingdale's, and then phoned. I was thrilled to hear from him because no one, not even my grandmother, had told me where he'd gone, and I had convinced myself that he'd fled the country, had landed in the Cayman Islands or Argentina or some other place where bad people typically hide out. I had images of him playing poker with Josef Mengele. To find out that he was still on U.S. soil, still in a place that Delta and United fly to, still in an area code I could dial directly, made his misdeeds seem less sinister, less global, and more personal. I don't know why I made this rather trivial distinction, but I did, perhaps because it was convenient, perhaps because I wanted to forgive him. *Of course* I wanted to forgive him: He was my father, the only one I had, and it seemed to me that having two parents was some kind of inalienable right. So he showed up outside of my high school to take me out to dinner one evening, we made up, hugged and kissed a lot, talked a lot, and then he returned to his happy hacienda on the Intracoastal and disappeared all over again.

But a few weeks before I left for college, I finally did go visit my father down in Florida, spent a long weekend lounging in the sun around his pool, making trips to Coconut Grove and Calle Ocho, doing the things I thought fathers and daughters were supposed to do together. I even talked to my stepmother a lot, told her how much her refusal to talk to me when I was little hurt, told her that it was very painful to be six years old, sitting on the same couch as she was, watching the same *Star Trek* episode as she was, and having her talk only to my father, refusing to acknowledge me. And she admitted that she resented my existence, confessed all her sins, said she was sorry for confusing me with my mother, sorry for hating the fact that my dad had this whole family life before she came along, and I really believed that we'd made some serious strides toward reparation. We had a lot of fun. I even thought that my father and I had achieved a break-through of sorts, that it would be possible for us to be close again. I actually wrote an article about it for *Seventeen*, talking optimistically about how we had gotten back together after several years of misunderstandings and anger. I thought it was going to be great.

Then he and my stepmother, in some new attempt at a bilateral relationship, came to see me up at school in the fall. He brought his Nikon and took pictures of me with all my friends in front of Matthews Hall, in front of the John Harvard statue, in front of Widener Library. He came with me to Justice class and pretended to be interested in Professor Sandel's neo-Kantian argument about why a town in Minnesota that wanted to ban pornography should be allowed to super-sede the First Amendment and do so. He had cappuccino and *medianoche* sandwiches with me at Pamplona, and let me in-troduce him to my various friends and acquaintances as they table-hopped and peddled gossip around the little café. He acted like a proud father visiting his lovely daughter at college. He behaved as if we were normal: Give us the right clothes and we could model for J. Crew.

But all I could think the whole time was, Who the fuck does this man think he is? He disappears from my life for four years—four fucking miserable years of insanity and depres-sion—and now I'm at Harvard, and everything seems fine. He thinks he can just come around here and get some photos of his perfect little Ivy League daughter as if none of that bad stuff ever happened. Where the fuck was he when I needed him?

I swore I'd never speak to him again. I swore that the

idea that I could ever forgive him, that we could ever be close again, was one of those dreams, just like the idea that I was going to get to Harvard and then everything would be perfect. This hatred overtook me, and I couldn't help myself. I wanted so much to forget the past, but it wouldn't go away, it hung around like an open wound that refused to scar over, an open window that no amount of muscle could shut. I remembered learning about the Doppler effect in high school science, about the paradoxical reaction between sound and space which causes a source of noise to get louder the farther away it moves from you. And that's how all this felt to me right then: The din of the anger I had for my father was even worse now that the actual problems were supposed to be receding into the past.

Nothing in my life ever seemed to fade away or take its rightful place among the pantheon of experiences that constituted my eighteen years. It was all still with me, the storage space in my brain crammed with vivid memories, packed and piled like photographs and old dresses in my grandmother's bureau. I wasn't just the madwoman in the attic—I was the attic itself. The past was all over me, all under me, all inside me.

And what I thought, every time I thought about my father, every time his name came up, was quite simply: I WANT TO KILL YOU. I wanted to be more mature, more reasonable, I wanted to have a big, fat, forgiving heart that could contain all this rage and still find room for kind, beneficent love, but I didn't have it in me. I just didn't.

Still, I sat dialing his number that night during finals, punching the digits into the receiver, the way a boomerang always returns to the same old place. It was a strange habit that I usually reverted to every time I felt lonely and depressed and certain that I had completely exhausted my resources—that is, I couldn't find any new man to get obsessed with. I'd call my dad thinking it would make me feel better. As I sat on the cold hardwood floor, listening to the phone ring, I was completely agitated, pushed to the quaking brink, hating my whole life, hating my father, and wanting to tell him, once and for all, as I never had before, just how much I hated him.

I called collect. "Hi, Elizabeth. What's up?" he asked after accepting the charges.

"Finals, you know, studying a lot. Nothing unusual. How about you?"

"Same old thing. I go to work, work all day, come home, watch TV, read, whatever."

"Oh." Strained silence. I didn't know what else to talk about, so I thought I'd mention some financial stuff. "Um, Daddy, listen. I'm wondering, did you ever get those doctor bills that I sent you? You know, for the psychiatric treatment that I needed in the fall when all that stuff was going wrong with all those people and everything. Remember?"

"Yeah, I got them."

"Well, but, you know, they keep billing me, since I guess you haven't paid them, and, um, you know, at the time, as I recall, you said you would. I mean, I think we even made some agreement through Dr. King, something about how you'd take them immediately to the insurance people at work and let them do the processing. Remember how you promised you'd do that?"

"I did then. But I won't now."

"But, Daddy, you promised." I started to think, Oh my God, I know I called looking for a fight, but I didn't think it would start so soon. I was expecting at least a little bit of friendly banter. Why was he already giving me a hard time about something that was so easy for him? All he had to do was sign his name on a couple of forms once a month, and this whole discussion could be avoided. Why did he always insist on turning every little thing into a hassle? Dealing with him was like dealing with a low-level bureaucrat whose only bit of control or power could be exercised by saying *no* to the people who came to him, the people who waited on line for hours, people who were not part of the reason he was so small and powerless, people who were small and powerless themselves. Jesus, the only contact my father had with his paternity was his ability to refuse to give me what I needed.

Fuck this. Fuck him. I can't believe I have to persist in this conversation.

"Daddy, I remember clearly your saying that since your insurance covered ninety percent of it anyway, you'd pick up the tab." I'd started seeing a psychologist in the fall, precisely because Daddy, via Dr. King, had agreed to pay the bills. If he hadn't done that, I wouldn't have gone in the first place, and now the cost had mounted into thousands of dollars, money I didn't have. "Daddy," I moaned, "you said you'd pay. I went into therapy only because I had a promise from you. I never would have otherwise."

"I said that then. And I made a promise. But you didn't keep yours," he said. "You've just been cold and nasty to me since our visit."

I felt the rage starting to creep out of me, absorbing and spreading like a tea stain on white cloth. "Who do you think you're talking to, Daddy?" I screamed. "What kind of idiot do you think I am?" I started to huff. "How dare you tell me that I've been cold and nasty to you, when it was you, not I, who went away without leaving a trace four years ago? What the fuck are you talking about?"

"Elizabeth, listen—"

"No, no, no. Fuck that. Fuck that shit. For once in your life, you listen to me. Because for four years, you have been disappearing on me over and over again, and then coming back with your apologies and your excuses, going on and on about how the lawyers told you that you should leave, and about how Mommy drove you away, and about how you had no choice. So you listen to me for once. Because I know that every time you've come back, I've been nice because you are my father and I love you and I wanted to have a daddy like everybody else did—"

I started to cry. I hadn't felt it coming. No rush, no warning. Suddenly my face was wet and my voice was receding from a yell to a whimper. "I wanted to have a daddy like everyone else. I just wanted to be normal. I just wanted my daddy back. I never fought with you. I never told you that I was angry at you for leaving. I was never cold and nasty because I didn't want you to go away again. I never had the guts. But then you'd go away anyway. And I would keep hoping that you'd come back again because all my friends had fathers, and they could say that their fathers were lawyers or businessmen or clothing manufacturers, but I never knew where you were or what you did, and instead of being angry at you, I wanted you to just be my daddy again."

"Elizabeth, listen—"

"No. I won't listen. Because for once you're going to get it right in your face and know how horrible you were! Just for once you're going to quit blaming everybody else and quit making me feel bad and just hear that the truth of the matter is that you're just a selfish horrible father and you left because you're irresponsible!"

Now he started to cry. "Elizabeth, don't you think I know that? Don't you think I've hurt for all those years that I couldn't live with you because your mother and I divorced and then I couldn't see you because I was so far away? Don't you think that was hard for me too? And I have paid. I have paid because I seem to have permanently lost the girl who was once my daughter who I loved."

"Words," I said. I had stopped crying. "It's all just words.

Goddamnit! You should know that actions speak louder than words. But I suppose when you're this lousy, words are all you've got left."

"Elizabeth, I don't know what to say." He was gasping. "You should know that this has ruined me too."

"Well, maybe," I continued. "But you had a choice. If you couldn't handle having a child, you shouldn't have had one. I didn't ask to be born. I got stuck." I knew this was a very manipulative thing to say and I didn't care.

"Elizabeth, I'm worried about you," he said, as if this would ameliorate my anger. I had never cried so hard. "Elizabeth, are you okay over there? Are you going to be all right?"

"Oh, fuck you! Stop trying to change the subject. Stop worrying about if I'm all right now. Obviously I'm not. But I wasn't all right then either. And you didn't care then, so why should you start now? It wouldn't be costing you a dime to do me this one favor and help me pay for therapy. I mean, obviously I needed help in the fall and I need it now. The only way I may ever be able to have a relationship with you ever again is if I get some help. And your response to all this is to not pay my medical bills even though it wouldn't cost you anything at all. Does that sound like what a good father would do?"

"Elizabeth, I'm sorry."

"You're always sorry," I yelled. "Instead of being sorry all the time, why don't you just be happy to be your rotten self?"

"But I'm not paying those bills. It's your mother's responsibility according to our divorce agreement."

"Oh Jesus, Daddy." More sobbing. "I could be dying here, going crazy, killing myself, and you'd still be standing there and saying that it's someone else's reponsibility to help me out, when you are the only one who is completely able to. Mommy is already overwhelmed with paying for school. But this is just the same old thing. This is awful."

"Elizabeth, I don't know what to say." He was crying pretty hard by now too. "I look back and see so many mistakes I've made and I feel powerless. I don't know how to correct what's already happened."

"You could start by paying for the psychiatric treatment I had in the fall and for me to maybe get some more help now, so that I can work out all this anger I feel for you."

"I won't do that," he said. "I already told you it's your mother's responsibility."

"Oh Jesus, Daddy. I give up. I can't listen to this anymore."

"What am I supposed to say?"

"Try, Have a good life. Because this is it for me."

Years later, thinking about this conversation, I will remember, as somebody very sagely said during the parricide trials of the Menendez brothers: *Anytime your kids kill you, you are at least partly to blame.*

On a Saturday night in May, I took some Ecstasy with Ruby to celebrate some minor triumph or other: At some point we'd decided we'd only do it if we could come up with a better reason besides that we're depressed and bored—and we ended up under a table at a party in the *Advocate* building, tying people's shoelaces together and watching them trip. We thought this was about the funniest thing ever until, suddenly, it started to seem hot and stuffy and claustrophobic and we just had to get out. That was how it was on Ecstasy: Every impulse quickly became an imperative, anything that might choke your buzz had to be destroyed, abandoned, shut up immediately. So we headed for the Adams House swimming pool, a creation of art deco decadence full of stone gargoyles and shiny tiles and stained-glass windows that had come to seem like our idea of paradise. Late at night, after whatever gatherings we'd been to, Ruby and I would retreat to the balmy blueness of the swimming pool, sit on the deck, and have our postmortem.

That night we talked and talked, babbled in Ecstasy incoherently until we could see the sun beginning to peek through the colored glass. All of a sudden, like everything else in my life that has seemed both catastrophic and unexpected, the humidity started to bother me. It started to bother me a lot. I was pretty sure I was going to suffocate. I wanted to ask Ruby if anyone had ever died from steam or precipitation or vapor or whatever the hell it was that was making me feel like we were trapped in a fucking cloud. My green wool dress itched against my sweaty flesh so much that I started to wonder if I didn't have chiggers or some other parasite crawling underneath my skin, and I remembered that the thing to do was put clear nail polish all over your body to suffocate the little critters. But standing here in this stuffy pool room, I reminded myself that it was I who was suffocating.

I stood up and stared into the aquamarine water that was flat and motionless. It felt like I was standing and looking down into that pool for hours, when really it was just minutes. I started to think that I might just like to fall into the water and drown. Die like a Rolling Stone, like Brian Jones. Die in a swimming pool and let my body float to the surface like William Holden's corpse in the opening shot of *Sunset Boulevard*. Go overboard like Natalie Wood, or drown deliberately like Virginia Woolf. Die young. Die glamorous.

Jesus Christ. Was I scared of suffocating to death or was I kind of wishing for it?

And how many times a day did death fantasies creep into my thoughts? So many times I had planned my own funeral, knowing for sure that any death at my age would be considered a tragedy, surely worthy of a full-length feature in some publication, maybe the *Boston Phoenix* or *New York*, where I'd been an intern during my senior year of high school. I knew perfectly how the story would go: She was so full of potential, Harvard, a dancer, a writer, blah blah blah. And then the reporter would try to figure out what it says about our society when a promising young person with so many options chooses to do herself in. I could see it all: My life would suddenly be infused with all sorts of symbolism and meaning that it simply did not have as long as I was alive. As long as I was alive, I'd be staring into swimming pools at daybreak, empty and aching.

But of course, I knew I'd stay alive. I knew that even if I jumped into the pool, I wouldn't have the guts to drown myself, though I am told that if you resist the natural urge to come to the surface for air, drowning is the least painful method of death that there is. Pain or no, I would most likely walk around in a suicidal reverie the rest of my life, never actually doing anything about it. Was there a psychological term for that? Was there a disease that involved an intense desire to die, but no will to go through with it? Couldn't talk and thoughts of suicide be considered a whole malady of their own, a special subcategory of depression in which the loss of a will to live has not quite been displaced by a determination to die? In those pamphlets that they give at mental health centers where they list the ten or so symptoms that would indicate a clinical depression, "suicide threats" or even simple "talk of suicide" is considered cause for concern. I guess the point is that what's just talk one day may become a real activity the next. So perhaps after years of walking around with these germinal feelings, these raw thoughts, these scattered moments of saying I wish I were dead, eventually I too, sooner or later, would succumb to the death urge. In the meantime, I could withdraw to my room, could hide and sleep as if I were dead.

I spent the next few days virtually comatose, ordering in food on the rare occasions when I was hungry. Ruby came and visited me when I didn't return any of her messages. Hadley, one of my floormates in Hurlbut who was starting her freshman year for the second time after being deferred by a suicide attempt and a stay at McLean, left me a card that said, "500,000 heroin addicts can't be wrong." It was the only laugh I'd had in a while. I panicked some about an exam that I had to take on Wednesday, but then I realized that I was at Harvard, the school with the all-purpose excuse system, so there was no reason to worry. That morning I went to U.H.S. and sicked out of the test, pleading mental problems. All I had to do was sign on the dotted line. (The staff never say no to anyone who doesn't want to take an exam for any reason, because the last time they did the guy killed himself.) When I explained to the nurse practitioner who handled my case that I'd been in therapy for a while but had run out of money and was all messed up again, she said I ought to go see a crisis management counselor at U.H.S. to help me sort out my immediate troubles.

"Mental health is on the third floor—" she started to say.

"I know where it is." I nodded. "Believe me, I know."

When I got upstairs, I was astonished by just how familiar the place had become, how accustomed I was to the magazines (*The Saturday Evening Post, National Geographic,* and other periodicals not even crazy people would want to read) and the bright orange plastic chairs in the waiting area. After a little while, I was called in by a woman doctor who had open office hours that morning. On her door it said HANNAH SALTENSTAHL, M.D. She sat in a swivel chair next to her large wooden desk, while I settled on a couch opposite her. The room was full of plants, posters, paintings, and Central American tapestries, which were supposed to make it less antiseptic and more cozy. I was used to therapists' offices after so many years in and out of them. They all looked the same. The decor that was meant to express individuality and comfort was actually just the universal look of a mental health practitioner's place of business.

I began with the beginning. I told her about my mother and father, I told her about coming to Harvard and all that it meant to me, I told her about my writing. Mostly I told her how lucky I was, how wonderful my life really was on paper, and how I would fall into these spells of depression for no reason, at the least likely times, times I ought to be happy. I told her about the black wave, that the feeling was literally physical, that the sensation was palpable, as if I'd drunk a bottle of tequila and taken some shitty windowpane and just lost my mind, that I was sure it was chemical. I wanted psychotropic drugs, I told her. I wanted her to prescribe me something that would make the rushes of misery stop. I wanted to break the black wave.

"Elizabeth," she said, "there is no pill in the world that's going to make you feel better. We have no way of measuring whether you have any sort of deficiency or not. The way we diagnose people for mental illness is purely anecdotal, and then we prescribe medications that we believe will suit the patient best by trial and error. Since there's not a blood test to detect depression or schizophrenia, we just have to figure out what works as well as we can. I see from your record that you've been here several times this year"—she said this while looking down at green and blue pages that seemed to be my file—"so I would love to help you if I could. But I assure you from what you've told me, and what I'm reading here, that your problem is not chemical."

"But isn't there some drug I can take so I can stop feeling unhappy at the most unlikely times?" I asked.

I was ready to scream, Give me lithium or give me death!

"I mean, I have every reason to be really happy and I'm not, and to me it seems that I must be chemically deficient. It's not normal to have these feelings for no reason. And I have violent mood swings too. One minute I'm ecstatic and the next I'm miserable. Maybe I'm a manic-depressive and maybe I need lithium. I keep thinking that. I keep thinking about all those famous manic-depressives like Anne Sexton who weren't diagnosed until late in life, so they suffered with these horrible highs and lows like I do, when lithium could have helped them all along." I was waiting for her to say something like, You're no Anne Sexton, but she didn't so I continued. "I just, Dr. Saltenstahl, I just don't want to end up a tragedy, and I think that's where I'm heading and I need help."

"Look, Elizabeth," she said, and her voice was telling me, My patience is infinite and unrelenting, and yet, it is still somehow limited, so just listen to me and understand what I'm saying. "It is not atypical of your generation to look for the chemical cure for everything. Wouldn't it be nice if we could all take happy pills and make the bad go away? We live in a drug culture, both legal and otherwise. But I'm not going to lie and tell you that some pill would help you when I know it wouldn't. From what you've told me about your parents, especially about your father, you've grown extremely detached over the years, as a defense mechanism. You don't need drugs, Elizabeth. What you really need is close, caring relationships. You need to trust somebody. You need to think people are okay."

"How can I think anything is okay when everything seems so horrible?" I started to sniffle. "I need help." Drugs! Please!

"I agree," she said, shaking her head. "You are obviously a very troubled person and it's going to take a lot of therapy to work through your problems." Deep breath, as if from exhaustion. "It takes a long time and a lot of thinking. It's

hard to change your life patterns. And you've been reinforcing your negative relationship habits for a long time now.
You say you've been depressed on and off since age eleven,
and you talk about the impact your father had on you by
leaving when you were fourteen. But I think the roots of
your depression go a lot deeper than the last eight years. They
start at early childhood and just get worse." She shook her
head in dismay and then smiled as a comforting afterthought.
"Look, I really am sorry that people over the years have hurt
you and turned you into a very depressed young woman,
because like you said, you have a lot to be happy and grateful
for. And I'm sure you will be eventually, but I'm afraid you've
got some hard times coming up. It's going to take a lot of
work for you to get better, and I don't know of any quick
fixes. It's going to be difficult."

"I know," I said. I started to cry, and she handed me a
Kleenex. "I really know."

A lot of good knowing did. Thanks to my father, I didn't
have the money to see a therapist—I was still paying off bills
from the fall—and Dr. Saltenstahl, who I liked very much in
spite of her refusal to prescribe any pills, was overbooked both
in her Harvard office and in her private practice. Besides, as
she pointed out, the people in the mental health department
at U.H.S. were meant to help students solve short-term problems only, and to refer them to long-term therapists if necessary. That was all she could do for me. She strongly urged
me to do whatever I needed to do to get into therapy with
a rigorous, smart doctor. Once again, I had to explain that
circumstances had conspired to make that just about impossible, unless I dropped out of school and worked full-time.
In the meantime, she felt compelled to remind me that if I
were ever feeling suicidal, I could go to the hospital emergency room and check myself in. It seemed that we were still

operating with the same old rules: Once you feel desperate enough to be institutionalized, there is help available, and insurance to cover the cost; until then, you're on your own, kid.

7

Drinking in Dallas

✳ ✳ ✳

I started out on burgundy
But soon hit the harder stuff.
Everybody said they'd stand behind me
When the game got rough.
But the joke was on me.
There was nobody even there to call my bluff.
I'm going back to New York City.
I do believe I've had enough.

BOB DYLAN
"Just Like Tom Thumb's Blues"

Summer of 1987. Dallas, Texas. The Oak Lawn section, to be precise. I have finished my sophomore year at Harvard. Somewhere down the road I managed to pick up the 1986 *Rolling Stone* College Journalism Award for an essay I wrote about Lou Reed for the *Harvard Crimson*, and now I have a summer job at the *Dallas Morning News* as an arts reporter.

This is exactly where I want to be: I have been enchanted with Texas forever, or at least ever since I first visited all my cousins down in Dallas when I was still a little kid. To me, Texas is big strong men in cowboy boots, rugged Thoreauvian individualists, mining for oil as if it were gold, which it kind of was at one time. And Dallas is just the commercial center of all that wildcat fuel, one big country club in one sprawling suburb where all the boys play football and all the girls dream of growing up and having plastic surgery. Brawny brothers and silicone sisters everywhere. I'm not crazy about that part of the culture, all the materialism and wealth wor-

ship, but I go to Dallas thinking it will be good for me: Untrammeled capitalists are too busy making and spending
money to be bothered with melancholia. Dallas, I believe,
will be so vibrant, so spanking new, so urban-cowboy rowdy,
so much the opposite of everything I associate with depression, so much brighter and shinier than all the dull darkness
of the Northeast.

Of course the reality when I arrive in Dallas is quite a
bit different. There is an oil glut, a concomitant real estate
glut, the economy is depressed (not as bad as Houston, everyone points out optimistically), and Big D is in kind of a
sorry state. Texas, in general, is *meant* to be rich, its entire
culture is about good old boys making it big quick, and Tex-
ans, particularly those in Dallas, don't seem able to handle
poverty gracefully. They still buy Baccarat crystal at Neiman
Marcus on Saturday, even if they just laid off two hundred of
their company employees on Friday. It's like watching a
grown man who's too proud to cry, who is desperately stifling
his tears, cry anyway.

Every house I pass seems to have a FOR SALE sign in
front, every apartment complex has a FOR RENT: ONE
MONTH FREE! posted at the entrance, and along the highways
there are tons of half-completed skyscrapers, pink granite and
silver glass affairs conceived in times of prosperity, which are
never going to be finished. Cranes and rubble everywhere:
They used to say that the Dallas mascot was a crane opening
its jaw to the blue skyline. This is nothing like the city I saw
when I was visiting my relatives who live in North Dallas
during the Republican Convention in 1984.

Dallas in 1987 is depressed and depressing.

Still, I am mysteriously happy here, at least at first. I live
in this grand and dreamy apartment that I'm subletting from
a city desk reporter who is trying to cohabit with her boyfriend. From the first time I looked at the place—which is

only $300 a month, even less than my weekly salary—I thought it was the most beautiful thing I'd ever seen, with French doors, a ceiling fan, a little porch lush with plants and flowers and greenery and a cast-iron and glass breakfast table, and the sort of vast, open kitchen area with blue and white Mediterranean tiles that made me want to put small spice plants and ivy by the sink and hang chimes by the window. The bathtub even had little feet, and its edges curved out like cappuccino froth overflowing a mug. I'd be living alone for the first time in my life, like a big girl, and I felt a certain joy at the idea of moving in. I kept walking through the rooms of this charming railroad flat, and thinking to myself, This will be mine, this will be mine, all mine. I felt like Audrey Hepburn in *Breakfast at Tiffany's*, the independent gal in New York, beaming to be on her own, smiling all the time as she strolls down Fifth Avenue; or like Mary Tyler Moore, throwing her hat, as if it were caution, to the winds of Minneapolis.

I love the apartment so much that sometimes I just want to roll around on the hardwood floors with rapt delight.

And much to my surprise, there's even kind of a counterculture in Dallas, a small one, but enough to entertain me for the summer. I end up spending a good deal of time in Deep Ellum, a warehouse district on the eastern edge of downtown where artists and musicians live in lofts with exposed pipes and whitewashed brick walls, where rock clubs are as spartan and vast as airplane hangars and all you can get to drink in them is beer in a can, where you can catch groups like Edie Brickell and New Bohemians playing outdoors at Club Dada once or twice a week. Deep Ellum seems so vital to me that it's almost corny. Here young people are trying to build a scene from scratch and live in an alternative way as if it were something brand-new. Which for them, of course, it is. Down in Deep Ellum, it's a bit like being lost in the sixties, not because all the kids who hang out there idolize or idealize that era and bring it back with retro touches, but because the Kennedy assassination so paralyzed the city that the sixties are hitting Dallas twenty years late.

I could have been happy in Dallas. Except for the car problem.

Having grown up in New York, I never learned how to drive, and the lessons I took in Cambridge in preparation for the summer didn't end up helping much when I slept through my road test. Without a driver's license, without a rental car, and without access to anyone else's car, I was going to have to do a lot of transit negotiating that summer. The *Morning News* would pay for my cabs when I was on assignment, but otherwise I would pretty much be at the mercy of strangers. I would have to schedule all my activities around other people. I would always leave things I enjoyed early or stay somewhere miserable late because I needed to go with my ride. I could never just run home for five minutes to change clothes or grab something the way anyone with a car could, so I had to plan my days carefully.

It sounds like a small price to pay, but that summer I came to understand why teenagers all over America associate a driver's license with freedom. I understood that without a car, I was basically trapped in Dallas. And when the big bad downs started kicking in, as I should have known they inevitably and eventually would, I'd find myself scared to death, alone in my apartment, with no way out.

For all of June and a lot of July, I was convinced that everything was really okay for the first time ever. I even started to think that I had recovered from my depression, that all I had ever really needed was a satisfying job that kept me busy, that all this sitting around and intellectualizing and analyzing and hypothesizing and contemplating and explicating and prognosticating all the time was the source of all my problems.

Semiotics, not a chemical imbalance, was killing me. I just needed to stop thinking so much and start doing.

I wrote like crazy, at least two or three reported pieces a week, sometimes more. I wrote like my life depended on it, which it kind of did. My editors were mystified by my productivity, thought I was mainlining copy or something. They rewarded me by letting me write odd and unconventional essays about art and feminism and Madonna and Edie Sedgwick, or anything else I could come up with, and then they'd stick them on the front of the Sunday section. They nominated me for awards from the Texas Newspaper Association and the Dallas Press Club. They paid for my overtime, which added up to so much money that I was practically doubling my salary (and it was costing them so much that after a while the assistant managing editor who oversaw my section of the paper suggested I take some comp days instead). My editors were pleased with my work and I was extremely prolific and conscientious. So they kind of let it slide when I started to crack.

Cracked in little ways. Walked into work at three in the afternoon on the grounds that I had to do some reading at home. Or had been up all night watching bands at the Theatre Gallery and couldn't function on no sleep. All of which was perfectly legit, no problem, my editor would say, so long as I didn't have to be in to go over some copy that day. But then, when I did arrive at my office, I spent most of my time returning personal phone calls or telling the other reporters about the latest man in my life, an ever-changing array of cowboys, restaurateurs, musicians, and college sophomores. I'd tear through them with such alarming alacrity that after a while I was dating brothers, cousins, entire families, it seemed. I found this all very amusing. I'd just blab and blab. People would look kind of entertained but mostly bewildered, as if to ask, Why is this girl telling us all this stuff? This is an *office*, people are trying to *work*, I think they sometimes wanted to say.

But no one really cared. I managed to meet all my deadlines, my work was always good, and, they figured, she's young, she's from up north where people chatter, no harm done. Even after everyone else left the office at 6:00, I would still be there for hours getting my pieces done since it was impossible for me to work when there were people around to talk to. Between so much writing and so much chatting, my weeks were too packed for me to notice my emotional state at all, except in passing blinks of fatigue.

But on weekends, with no exigencies of the moment beckoning at my head, I realized that I was all alone in the great state of Texas and all alone in the world. Even the brief, two-day gap in activity was enough time for that old ugly feeling, that familiar black wave, to start creeping up on me, threatening to drag me away. Since I slept so little Monday through Friday, you'd have thought that I'd appreciate the days off to catch up, but I could barely sleep anyway, and my nights passed fitfully. I was tired all the time, but unable to find relief. It was like being on cocaine after the trippy effect has worn off and all that's left is a wired feeling that keeps you staring at the ceiling all night, unable to doze. The only difference was this was not the aftereffect of some coke—this was me. So I filled up the hours as best I could. No one else wanted to surrender a Saturday to cover a day of heavy metal that was known as the Texxas Jamm, so of course I expressed my willingness to review Poison, Tesla, and the rest of the motley assortment of bands that would be playing at the football stadium. No one else wanted to spend July Fourth in Waxahachie at Willie Nelson's Picnic, so I did my civic duty and accepted the assignment. Pain in the ass though I was, who could really fault a girl who'd saved them from having to cover these tawdry and embarrassing bits of Texas culture that only a Yankee could appreciate?

To a certain extent, anyone who's alone and new to an area would be inclined to do a lot of running around, and at first I thought all my manic energy was the result of simple curiosity and the novelty of Dallas. But I was hardly a stranger in a strange place: I'd spent a lot of time in Texas when I was growing up, I'd traveled from one end of the state to the other, I had family in Dallas, I knew the town pretty damn well, and I could very easily have spent weekends in the peaceful company of my relatives, eating barbecue and going to the mall. Sometimes I did do that. But it was never pleasant for me. I was so nervous all the time, always feeling like there was something I should be doing but wasn't, always feeling at the mercy of something that felt like a hive of bees buzzing in my head.

Once I woke up at three in the morning, but without my glasses on I mistook the three on my digital clock for an eight. In fear of being late for—for whatever—I charged out of bed, jumped in the shower, dressed, made myself up, drank coffee, and ate Cocoa Krispies, and only as I grabbed my handbag to walk out the door did I notice that the sky was dark, it was the middle of the night, there was no need to rush. And it's not exactly like I had to punch a time clock. When I got back into bed, I laughed to myself a little bit, and then I just thought, This is crazy. What's happening to me? I've got all this energy, not the refreshing, delightful kind but the edgy anxious type, and not a damn thing to do with it. If the editors of the *Dallas Morning News* decided one day that I had to write the entire contents of the newspaper by myself, I still wouldn't be busy enough to satisfy this enormous, deleterious need I have to keep moving. There will always be this deficit, this flabby remainder of self hanging over me, demanding more attention than I and seventy-two other people put together could possibly satisfy. What I wouldn't do to be Alice climbing through the looking glass, taking one of those pills that makes you small, so small. What I wouldn't do to be less.

And I started to think, Damn, I need medicine. I need something reining in all this thinking. Because I'm going to go crazy like this. I was almost twenty years old, which is often the age that people with bipolar illness experience their first manic episode, so maybe that's what was happening to me. When I wasn't working, I was out partying, dating sixteen different men at once, never sleeping at night, gulping Jolt cola and snorting speed for breakfast so I could get through the rest of the day. I figured out that I could manage my moods fairly well if I stuck to a rigorous chemical routine of beer and wine in the evenings, followed by mornings of major uppers.

Drinking in Dallas was a lot more fun than it had ever been anywhere else, although I couldn't say why. Perhaps it was because I took to hanging with some hard-news reporters who tended to hard-drink with relish. In fact, to talk to them, you'd almost think that alcoholism was the sign of a journalist doing his job well, a sign of someone who'd seen the blood, the white outlines, the body bags, all the gore of a triple murder, and drank to clear his head of all the ugly he was forced, and perversely delighted, to see. But the variety of alcohol-related experiences also excited me. At the time, Corona beer was available only in the Southwest, and having a bottle with a lime squeezed into it was such a novelty to me, a brilliant admixture of a real drink and a simple brew. Boilermakers—a shot of bourbon, preferably Maker's Mark, quite literally thrown glass and all into a stein of beer—were another new discovery. Getting a hold of some speed—whether it was methamphetamine or Dexedrine or Benzedrine—was a pretty easy task because the drug scene in Dallas was so clean cut. It seemed like everyone lived next door to some nice collegiate dealer who was putting himself through Southern Methodist University selling plants, pills, and powders, or knew someone else who did. But usually all it took was all the caffeine and sugar provided in Jolt to get me through the day, so the cycle of up and down could be maintained cheaply and legally.

One night, I planned to interview the Butthole Surfers after they played a gig down in Deep Ellum. As it happens, they were leaving for a European tour the morning after they played Dallas and decided that rather than get only a couple of hours of sleep after the show, they'd just not sleep at all. So I stayed up with them, smoking their weed, sipping on Coronas with lime, hearing stories about their pit bulls, hearing about how they had an indirect sexual encounter with Amy Carter by rubbing their private parts on her suitcase when they played at Brown University, hearing about how one of their former drummers is now a bag lady living in San Francisco's Golden Gate Park, hearing about how they got the name the Butthole Surfers, and realizing that these guys were the real-life embodiment of the movie *Spinal Tap*. I learned that they had once been called the Winston-Salems and now occasionally played local bar gigs under the name the Jack Officers.

I was so amused that I just kept getting more and more stoned and drunk, and the last thing I remember before I went home to shower and change my clothes so I could go back to the office is standing behind the club, in a back alley, talking to the guitarist, who was, I thought at the time, the cutest thing alive, with sweet brown eyes and a compelling smile, the combination of which, when he looked at me so directly and soberly even though he'd smoked even more pot than I had, made me want to do anything, anything for him. Never mind that I was feeling stoned and sensual and was dying to take all my clothes off, even back there, standing next to the junkyard, the site of new construction, part of the gentrification process, and surrounded by nothing but the night. We started to kiss, his shirt came off, and pretty soon his hands dug under my blouse, rubbing my breasts as his finger made circles around my nipple. And I reached into his pants, touched him, touched his half-flaccid penis that got harder as I held onto it, and suddenly I realized that I didn't want to do this.

It hadn't even been a year since I lost my virginity to a recent Yale graduate who I'd met at the *Rolling Stone* College Journalism Award luncheon. It hadn't even been a year since I decided that my mouth was getting tired and chapped from giving so many blowjobs, that it was time to start having sex like a normal nineteen-year-old. It hadn't even been a year since my complete initiation into sexual activity, and I was not ready to start screwing around with a virtual stranger— with whom, I might add, it was unethical for me to be carrying on—in some Dallas back alley. Somehow, I had this moment of truth, and I felt certain that I didn't want this, didn't want to live this life, had to get out of there right then. So I pulled my hands away from his fly, pulled my shirt back on, and started to run, but the thing was, I couldn't run anywhere. I had to call a taxi first. And I thought to myself, You know, this sucks. It sucks when you can't make a clean getaway.

And I felt that something was very, very wrong. What had I wanted from that guy, anyway? Why had I led him outside in the first place? This seemed to be a routine for me, getting started on sexual encounters and not only stopping them, but actually fleeing from the room as if in shame or in danger, realizing that *I just don't want to be there*, that I felt trapped and cramped. I wanted so badly to lose myself in sex, to be thoroughly slutty and have one zipless fuck after another. I wanted to be a wild thing. But in the end, I couldn't ever go through with it because it's never like that, there was no pleasure for me in being an easy lay. Fast, cheap sex was no fun at all. My body and mind are just too complicated. I'd seen movies like *9½ Weeks*, and I envied the Kim Basinger character and the way she could achieve a full—even multiple—orgasm while standing in the rain with her back against a brick wall in a dark cul-de-sac as street thugs chased after her and Mickey Rourke with knives and guns, as a stray cat strutted by with a dead rat in its mouth. How I would have loved to be one of those women who got excited over such excitement. But frankly, given that same situation, I'd be wanting an umbrella, I'd want to get indoors, I'd want to dry my cold, chafing feet and hands, and sex would be almost unthinkable.

I had tried so hard for so many years to turn all my despair into sexual abandon, I wanted so much to stop being me and start being someone else's toy, but I didn't have it in me. Those early encounters with Abel when I was twelve were the best experiences I'd ever had. He'd been so sweet to me, and he'd taught me about the ways my body could give and receive pleasure, he showed me so much, and he made me so happy. When I was with Abel, I felt like ice cream in a bowl, melting away, knowing that soon I would be completely gone, but if it made him as happy to lick me up as I felt being consumed, that was just fine. It hadn't ever been that way again.

My God, I thought, as I waited in Deep Ellum for a taxi. My God, how I need a drink.

When I finally drift off to sleep, time disappears. I can't remember if the Butthole Surfers interview was yesterday or the day before or today, if the Suzanne Vega story was written last week or last month or last year or just yesterday, or when the hell I went to the rap concert, because it feels like ages ago. Is tomorrow Saturday or is it Monday? Do I have to get up in the morning or can I sleep? Will anyone even know the difference? I can be as fucked up as I like, it seems, as long as I get my work done, and I always do, so everyone writes everything else off to hormones.

No one in Dallas really cares about me. I'm a stranger in town and on earth. No matter how I tell myself I am familiar with this place, it isn't true. I'm a stranger wherever I go because I'm strange to myself. My mind just goes off doing its own thing, never consulting me at all about whether it's all right to feel this way or that. I am constantly standing several feet away from myself, watching as I do or say or feel something that I don't want or don't like at all, and still I can't stop it. The closest I get to keeping myself in line is when I drink. With enough wine, I can even sleep at night. I wonder what I will have to do to convince some medical doctor that I am really and truly imbalanced, that there's no other explanation for the way my head feels all the time, for the way I feel like one of those souvenir plastic domes that are full of glitter which you get at Disney World or at truck stops, the kind that makes snow when you turn it over. That's what it's like in my head all the time, constant snow, constant weather patterns of all sorts—blizzards, cyclones. I am the fucking Wizard of Oz. I can't go on like this much longer. Why won't any of the doctors help me? I've gone to so many, and they all say, You need love. Or, You need to talk this through. Don't they see that all their advice may be well intentioned but in the meantime I'm falling, I know it, I am.

By the time my mother came to visit, it seemed perfectly normal to me to spend the whole week boozing around and giving over entire weekends to unwinding by the pool at my cousins' house. I stopped noticing that I often forgot about eating. When my mother was shocked by how skinny I'd gotten, I was shocked to find out this was the case.

I was even more surprised to find out that she wanted

to throw me a birthday party at my cousins' house. It all seemed like an okay enough idea to me, although if I had thought about it, I'm sure I'd have realized that it was a big mistake. My mother, consummate mother that she is, would be incapable of keeping it simple, would inevitably spend hours making the right marinade for the barbecue chicken, her own special honey mustard sauce for sandwiches, and the perfect pear tarts and apple crisp and birthday cake for dessert.

She would, in other words, go through hours and hours of trouble, when the truth was that I probably would have just as soon spent my birthday with my friends, all of whom lived near downtown like I did and never went to far North Dallas, where my family lived, for any reason. And as it turned out, I had so much trouble giving people directions to my cousins' house, that after a while I just decided it would be a small affair, I could catch up with my pals later.

My birthday fell on a Friday, and my boss decided that my whole department would go out for drinks after work to celebrate. It had been a miserable day. Around the office, very few people even knew it was my birthday, which wouldn't have been alarming except that I spent so much time telling so many people brutal, minute details of my life that I felt like everyone knew me better than they really did. Because, of course, what I was giving all my coworkers was just schtick, false intimacy at best. They'd have gotten to know me better if I'd sat quietly by myself and never said a word. I got birthday calls from people in Cambridge and Berkeley and New York (my ex-boyfriend Stone forgot it was my birthday but phoned to let me know he'd slept with Ruby while he was on acid and he hoped I'd forgive him), but the only person in Dallas who bothered to check in with me that day was my mother. Why did it always seem as if the fates had conspired to make me feel like she was the only one on earth who loved me?

I sat at my desk depressed all day, and it amazed me that even though I burst into tears no one asked what was wrong. I guess they all felt that it was somehow none of their business.

At the end of the day, when the other people in my department came to gather me so that we could go to Louie's for drinks, I was relieved. I spent a couple of hours at the bar drinking beer with bourbon and gin with tonic, chasing tequila-lime-salt shots with Cinzano and lemonade, and time just slipped through the pouring drinks. By the time I finally realized that I had to get to my cousins' house for my party, that I was already late, no one much felt like driving that far out.

Car problems again, I thought. But instead of getting up and calling a taxi, I ordered another drink. I asked for a Glenlivet straight up, told the waiter to make it a double and save himself a trip. I didn't realize that I'd already had a few too many until I stood up and felt myself stumble as if I were walking on a very unstable rowboat that was starting to rock. I grabbed onto the nearest wall, collected myself, headed for the pay phone, and tried to convince my cousin Bruce that I was trapped, had no way of getting to the house, couldn't he come and pick me up. He was my age, after all. Surely he'd understand about getting too fucked up before you have to face your family, surely he'd want to help me out of a bind. But instead of answering, he just started yelling, "Where the fuck are you? Your mother has been slaving in the kitchen all day so she could throw a party just for you, and where are you?"

"Oh, Bruce," I answered. "Oh, Bruce, I'm stuck. I can't stand straight I'm so drunk. I feel so bad. She never should have done this. Bruce, please come get me. Please."

"No way. You got yourself into this, you can get yourself out of it. Call a cab and get your ass up here now. I offered to pick you up earlier, but it's late now, so hit the road."

"Bruce, I don't think I have enough money—"

"Get someone to lend it to you, then, but just get here before your mother is really upset."

When I stumbled into my cousins' house at 9:30, I was three hours late for my own party, and the first thing I did was run to the bathroom and throw up. All of my mother's friends and business associates who lived in North Dallas were in attendance, and my mother was mortified.

There were chicken cutlets and birthday cake and blowing out the candles and presents and a toast to the birthday girl and all that other stuff, but we had to do it all fast because it was so late. I kept wishing I could leave or wishing I'd gotten there much earlier or something. My mother looked so sad and sorry the whole night. I kept walking up to her and trying to hug her, to thank her, to explain that I was just depressed and I'd been drinking, and given that combination I couldn't control my own behavior, but it was useless. She kept pushing me away, telling me she'd had it with me, telling me that she couldn't believe what a rotten child I was.

And I kept saying, Mommy, Mommy, I'm so depressed, I'm losing my mind, please don't push me away from you. And she would say, I can't help it, *you've* pushed me away from you.

And half of me thought, I've really fucked up this time, and the other half was a little angry at my mother for going through all this trouble for me when I hadn't asked her to and yet again putting me in a position where I could only be the ungrateful child. When all the guests finally left, my mother cried on the deck by the pool, and I cried on the living room sofa, and my cousin Bruce sat down next to me and put his arm around my shoulder, and I said, "We're quite a pair, my mother and I, aren't we?"

"Look, the only reason I'm being halfway nice to you is

that it's your birthday, and that I do think that she shouldn't have done all this for you, but you really are a shithead."

"I know."

It was always this way though: I spent most of my life trying to please my mother, and instead I just disappointed her.

Bruce drove me back to my house in Oak Lawn. We rode together in his father's Porsche in silence. It wasn't until I walked in the door that he screamed out his window, *Hey, cousin, are y'all gonna be all right?* As I reassured him with some vigorous nods, I went into the vestibule and checked my mailbox. And there, along with an L. L. Bean catalogue and a bill from Lone Star Gas, were three birthday cards, all from my father. My father whom I hadn't spoken to in at least a year.

How the hell, I wanted to know, had he gotten my address? How did he know that I was in Texas at all? And why did he have to disturb me on my already disturbing birthday?

I opened the cards when I got upstairs. The envelopes were numbered so I could read them in order, and all of them were about how his love for me stayed strong and steady even though we were apart. All of them were Hallmark cards with Rod McKuen-type poems on them that you would send to your long lost lover, not your daughter.

And I thought: This is twisted.

Maybe it's not that unusual anymore for entire families to be estranged from each other, maybe the way my father disappeared without a trace for so long is just how it goes, and maybe it makes perfect sense that he would somehow find me here in Texas so he could send me sentimental, romantic cards on my birthday, addressing me as his "Little One." But if this is the way things are going to have to be, then I reject this life. And even if every family on earth were like mine, if divorce were mandatory, if custody battles were routine, if everyone's mother was suing everyone's father and vice versa, it wouldn't make mine any less twisted. And it wouldn't make me feel any better to be sitting in my apartment in Dallas watching a three-inch palmetto crawl down a wall, so big and ugly I don't want to get close enough to kill it, just hoping it'll have its space and let me have mine because, I think, I'm going to crash.

But I was too upset to rest, too drunk to drink anymore, too unhappy not to, so instead I walked out of my apartment and out of my house, and headed down Oak Lawn Avenue, fast and solid, strutting in my blue jeans and pointy cowboy boots like a woman with a mission. Of course, I had nowhere to go. I was a pedestrian in a city where only the indigent and insane walk anywhere at all, but I kept on going because the idea of movement, the idea that I could walk wherever I wanted to, that I was free within my own body, was liberating enough to take the edge off how shitty I felt.

And without knowing why, I found myself walking toward the *Morning News* music critic's house, which was right near mine. I kind of had a crush on Rusty, and at any rate he was good to talk to, so I figured that visiting him was a good idea. But when I arrived at his cute little saltbox house, which was right next door to a gas station and opposite a Sound Warehouse, the lights were out and his Suzuki jeep was gone. But I rang the bell and banged on the door anyway. I pounded and pounded and pounded as if the power of my fist knocking on wood could conjure Rusty back from wherever he was. It was my birthday, after all, or at least it had been until about an hour ago. It was my birthday, and Rusty ought to have been around for me if I wanted him to be, goddamnit.

I just kept pounding for at least ten minutes, unaware or indifferent to the noise my banging was making, until the gas station attendant finally walked over to see what was wrong.

And I looked up at his face, his simple face that was questioning mine, wondering what a girl like me was doing throwing herself at this door, and all I could do was cry.

And something about him seemed so nice. Oh God! Oh God! I screamed. Everything is wrong, everything is so wrong.

He didn't really know what to do. He drove me home, and all the while I cried and told him that I thought I was having a breakdown. He was silent, and for a moment I worried that he was maybe going to want to come upstairs with me, that maybe he would rape me, that I didn't know who he was, what his name was, but I was crying to him which might have suggested a familiarity that I had no desire to achieve at that moment. And then I realized how silly I was being: Women weeping mournfully for the dead or happily at a wedding can be quite attractive, but a hysterical girl, a girl writhing in your car with her face bloated and red from crying, her hair springing out of her head from the humidity—no guy wants to get into this girl's pants.

And indeed I arrived home safely, drank another bottle of Chardonnay, and fell restlessly to sleep.

In the morning I woke up to my mother standing over my bed—I must have left the front door open—with a piece of paper she wanted me to sign. It said something to the effect that she would pay for my college tuition, because that was her obligation to me, but nothing more. The only reason I knew what this piece of paper said was that she read it to me. I was too passed out to see, but when I heard what she was saying, all I could do was stumble to the bathroom and throw up. I was so nauseated and hung over. When I wobbled back into my bedroom and flopped back into my bed, all I could say was, "Excuse me."

I looked at her and I figured that I'd better just sign this paper, that she would probably forget about it by next week anyway. "Listen, Elizabeth," she said sternly. "You have pushed me over the edge here. All I've ever done was love you, the only reason I threw you a birthday party was to make you happy, and you treat me so shabbily." She started to cry. "How can you treat me this way? What have I ever done to you?"

"Oh, Mom." I stood up and tried to hug her, but she pushed me away.

"No," she said. "I'm not going to be swayed by you. I'm just going to give you a piece of advice because I love you and you're still my child. I think you're an extremely troubled person and have been for a long time, and you resent me for whatever reasons. And I think that if I were you, I would just stay here in Dallas, don't go back to school, earn your own living, and spend your money on therapy. You like your job and people here seem to like you, so why don't you just stay, take time off from Harvard. Because"—she got all choked up—"I can't afford to send you to Harvard and put you in therapy, and I can see that all the years that you haven't been in therapy have really taken a toll. I look at you now, and I see a person really in trouble."

She headed for the door, and I wanted to stop her, but I felt too weak, and this was all too much first thing in the morning. The last thing she said before she left was, "I just want you to know that if you decide to leave Dallas at the end of the summer, that's fine. But you're paying for your ticket home and there will be a strict code of behavior observed once you get back."

Later that week, a producer for *Oprah!* called to ask if I would appear on a show they were doing about fathers who abandon their children. She had dug up the article I'd written for *Seventeen* by looking in *The Readers' Guide to Periodical Literature*, under "Divorce." The piece was mildly optimistic, suggesting that my father and I had in fact renewed our relationship. Since then, the preponderance of evidence had shown that my father and I were doomed never to have a relationship again. Why go on TV and talk about this instance of ugliness in the world? But the producer asked me if I would be willing to anyway, and it sounded like it could be fun, so I suspended my better judgment, and said, Sure, why not?

Mostly I was thinking it would be fun to go to Chicago and get the hell out of Dallas for a couple of days. My boss thought it was a great idea, said she'd give me the day off, told me that everyone would watch the show together when it was aired, and everyone around the newspaper seemed to think it was a good thing to do. My friend Tom, a city desk reporter, thought that maybe somebody would even see me on TV and find my story compelling and want to turn it into a movie or something.

That clinched it for me: I thought if I could become a movie, if I could disappear into celluloid, I could stop being me for a while. *I would do anything not to be Elizabeth.* Of course, nothing had worked so far. Going to Harvard, writing articles, working at the newspaper—I'd done all these things and still, somehow, I kept being me. Which is why I started to think that maybe I didn't want to be on *Oprah!* after all. It was too much the sort of thing I would do: Take a sad private matter, give the facts in technicolor detail to perfect strangers, and thus relieve myself of my life. And then later, I would feel cheap and empty, deeply dissatisfied, like a verbal slut, the girl who'd give it all away to just any old anybody. So maybe I wanted to reclaim my life, make it private, make it mine. Maybe, just maybe, if I lost the urge to tell all to all, maybe that would be behavior befitting a happy person and maybe then I could be happy.

The key to happiness, I decided, was *not* to appear on *Oprah!*

After all, I was the girl who lost her virginity and then gave consent when my friends decided to throw a party celebrating the occasion. It seemed like a funny idea, and heaven knows I'd waited plenty long enough. The Macintosh-printed invitations read, "Please come to a seminal and groundbreaking party in honor of Elizabeth Wurtzel," and inside was a picture of a flower that had dropped from its stem. Although the idea was supposed to be subtle, everyone who came to the party knew the occasion. A lot of girls walked up to me to tell me it was wild—totally wild—that I did something like this, that they'd wished they'd had a party when they'd first done it, but many more people thought I was very weird.

Including the guy whom I'd actually slept with, who couldn't make sense of why I'd taken this private matter between me and him and turned it into a public spectacle. And I couldn't answer. All I knew, and I couldn't say this to him as we spoke long distance between my dorm room in Cambridge and his apartment in Washington, D.C., was that here was something that meant a lot to me, the one remnant of my body that I was saving for true love or for a better time when I wasn't depressed and when my relationships with men were more than just random, desperate gropings for something that didn't hurt the way the rest of life did. And instead, in truth, I gave it away.

Gave my virginity to a guy who didn't really care about me very much, who was asking me now how I could take this private matter and turn it public, but the truth was it had never been really private. He never really knew me, knew the inside of me, not just my flesh but the soft center deep down that no one gets to see. So as far as I was concerned, he had invaded my body with his, and it felt good and it felt interesting, but in the end it wasn't something private no matter how I tried to convince myself. It never meant shit. I wanted, so badly, for sex to happen the right way with the right person at the right time in the right place, until, one day, during my sophomore year of college, I discovered that the enchanted situation I was waiting for didn't exist for me. So I decided just to love the one I was with.

I gave it away.

But my dad and I—that was different. I decided within a matter of hours after accepting the *Oprah!* invitation that there was no way I could appear. My father, and whatever was left of my relationship with him, was still mine. And I would not give that away. But by the time I got around to calling Diane, the producer, she had already decided that what she really wanted—wouldn't this be great?!—was to have me and my father appear on *Oprah!* together so that we could share both of our perspectives "to help illuminate the issues and achieve a better understanding of what causes men to abandon their children." And as she proposed this idea to me, I kept pointing out that I didn't even talk to my father and had no idea of his whereabouts, though based on the postmark on my birthday cards, I suspected he was somewhere in Virginia. "That's no problem," Diane told me. "We have people who can track him down so that we can stage a reunion on television. How long did you say it's been since you've spoken to him?"

She didn't get it. Or maybe she did and decided to proceed anyway. After all, it was her job to get people to discuss their private lives publicly. The point that I failed to convey is that there was no way that I was going to see my father for the first time in years on national television. "I think that's a terrible idea," I said.

At first, I was shocked that Diane could even suggest this family reunion, and then I realized that this is just the way of the world, or at least the way of *fin de siècle* America. Not only would the next revolution be televised, but so would every other little stupid thing. It was already happening: Television reunions between adopted children and their birth parents; encounters between a husband, his mistress, and his wife; discussions among killers on death row—in irons, via satellite—and the families of their victims; confrontations between incest survivors and their abusive relatives; meetings between a corrupt plastic surgeon and the women whose faces he deformed with wrinkle-reducing silicone injections that turned out to be toxic; a priest, a rabbi, a monk, and a minister (no, this is not the beginning of a bad joke) who have slept with members of their congregations. You could see all these events on simple, old-fashioned network television, all in a single day.

For so many people, or at least for the guests who were fodder for these shows, nothing seemed too sacred for the camera's lens. There was even a computer database listing the names of people who wanted to appear on talk shows, giving descriptions of their particular quirks, eccentricities, and handicaps. Many of the people who consented to talk about their private lives in front of millions of television viewers would say that they were sharing their stories as a way to comfort fellow sufferers, to raise public awareness, to give a voice to their pain. None of them would ever admit that it was all about ratings and voyeurism and lurid, grotesque curiosity. None of them would be able to see me and my friends sitting in our dorm rooms watching these shows in the late afternoon lull, laughing at their kitsch value. They'd all believe that what they were doing was good. In fact, Diane had originally tried to sell me on the whole *Oprah!* appearance by saying that it was a public service. When it was just me, I almost bought it; once she started talking about getting both me and my dad, I knew this was all just show biz, and it made me sick.

Still, Diane called me, day after day, and in the evenings

at home. I didn't have an answering machine, so that weekend I went to my cousins' house to escape the ring of the telephone, the awful sound of the bell that was not my mother calling to say she still loved me, was not some man I was wild for calling to tell me how much he cared, but just a woman I'd never met and never would wanting to know if my personal life could be exploited for her purposes.

The rest of the summer, what a mess. I get myself involved with Jack, a police-beat reporter who works from four in the afternoon until midnight, so that means that I end up staying up the rest of the night to drink with him. We're so drunk, we barely even fuck. I spend a lot of time miserable and vomiting. I go through a tube of toothpaste a day. I realize that no matter how hard I try, I will never be an alcoholic. A drug addict, maybe. But all drinking ever does is make me puke.

Every night, I sit in my apartment waiting for the clock to strike twelve, petrified that Jack won't call me, that he won't want to see me, that he'll run off with someone else, certain that if such a thing does happen, I will have no choice but to climb into my little old-fashioned bathtub and burgundy-stain the hot water with blood from my own wrists. That's how desperate Jack makes me feel. He makes me feel like suicide. I barely know him, our whole affair amounts to only a couple of weeks, but I am positively obsessed from the start.

Sometimes as I lie on the floor in the dark by the phone waiting for his call, I try to figure out what in the hell has gotten into me. Why am I so afraid of not hearing from him? It wouldn't be so bad. I could get some sleep for a change. I could get started on reading one of the tomes I'd schlepped down from Cambridge in preparation for my junior tutorial. I could try The Second Sex, *I could plow through* A Vindication of the Rights of Women, *I could figure out how the hell to free myself from this enslavement to men. Of course, Simone de Beauvoir was basically a fool for Sartre, and I seem to recall learning that Mary Wollstonecraft was over her head for—who was it?—John Stuart Mill, I think. But Jack is no Jean-Paul. In fact, if it weren't such a devastating thought, I could probably admit that Jack is no nothing. Pick a man, any man. Every guy I fall for becomes Jesus Christ within the first twenty-four hours of our relationship. I know that this happens, I see it happening, I even feel myself, sometimes, standing at some temporal crossroads, some distinct moment at which I can walk away*—just say no—and keep it from happening, but I never do. I grab at everything, I end up with nothing, and then I feel bereft. I mourn for the loss of something I never even had. I am a sick, sick girl.

God, do I ever want my mommy. Of course, my mom doesn't talk to me lately. It's just me, Jack, and the bottle.

One Saturday, Jack and I are supposed to see a matinee of The Big Easy. *He's supposed to call but never does. Hours go by, I can't leave my house, there's no answer on his phone, and I feel that exact desperation that I had feared night after night. There are a million things I can do to pass the time, but I feel so trapped and frightened, too agitated to read or do anything useful, so I find the only alcohol that's left in the house, some really nasty smelling rum, and figure it's never too early to get started. And then I remember that Globe, this guy I know who's in an industrial/rap band and dates the police commissioner's daughter and also deals on the side, has left a whole stash of psilocybin mushrooms in my closet. So I eat them. All of them. Maybe ten grams, I don't know. By the time the stuff kicks in, I might as well be on Pluto.*

I call all the people I know and talk to their answering machines. I go to the Sound Warehouse and buy—heaven help me—four Grateful Dead albums. I find Rusty and get stoned with him, even though I'm already 'shrooming. Then I decide that I really must walk. I walk for miles and hours, all the way to the slums of South Dallas, almost over to Oak Cliff. I walk through Deep Ellum, and even though I can't stop laughing and all the faces around me look like claymation, I manage to eat chicken-fried steak and biscuits with cream gravy at some little diner. I walk some more.

I inadvertently wander into a New Bohemians concert at a club near Grant Park. I hear Edie's voice, its lovely lilt, singing about circles and cycles and spinning round and round. I sit in the bleachers, I daze and doze to the sound of a voice and guitars and mandolins and percussions. I fade into what feels like thousands of strings. This is the happiest moment I've had all summer, this is the best place to be right here and right now, if only my whole life could be words and music, if only everything else could slip away. No Jack, no mother, no work, no play, nothing at all. Why does every little thing, even the happy things, inevitably turn into a great big encumbrance? If only everything could be as pure as this moment. If only I could freeze into this place forever.

And then Edie starts singing "Mama Help Me," all this stuff about crazy people, mean people, street people, and her voice is suddenly harsh, I am jolted out of my reverie, I remember who I am: I am the girl who took several times the normal dose of psilocybin mushrooms several hours ago, all because some guy I barely know didn't call when he said he would. I am the girl who has disappointed her mother. I am the girl out of perspective. I am the girl who needs to go home. "Where will I go when I cannot go to you?" Edie sings. "Mama mama m-m-mama help me, mama mama mama tell me what to do."

God, do I need help, I think, as I leave this outdoor club, this hippie version of a theater in the round. I get into a taxi—for once one is waiting, maybe there is a God—and as we drive along Central I feel wetness dripping down my face. Where is this coming from? I realize, sitting in the back seat, that I am weeping, that so much salt and water is pouring from my tear ducts, but because I am tripping I can't feel myself crying. At best, I can watch myself, sit alongside this vacant corpse of mine, and watch the roll of tears, but there is no sense of release because there's no one inside. I'm gone. Knock-knock? I've disappeared. I've come so close from so far, I hide behind this window and look at myself, look at a life I'd rather not see.

★ ★ ★

When I get home, David, the music critic from the *Dallas Times Herald*, is waiting on my stoop. Apparently, I'd had a date to go see Billy Squier with him several hours earlier that evening. When he couldn't find me after I'd left several messages on his answering machine reporting that I was "bottoming out," "losing it," and other such things, he got worried. He even called Rusty to see if he knew where I'd gone. When he couldn't find me, he went to the show but kept calling, and then after he'd filed his review, he drove around Deep Ellum looking for me. He kept bumping into people who'd seen me here and there, but he seemed to keep missing me. So he decided to wait until I got home.

"Are you all right?" he asks.

I am standing in front of him crying. "Do I look all right?" I ask in response.

"Not particularly, but one never knows with you."

"Fuck you!" I scream. "Fuck everybody! What do you mean, 'One never knows with you'? I'm a person like everybody else! I get upset like everyone else! When I cry, it's the same as when anyone else does. It means I'm hurting. Goddamnit, David! I'm really hurting. I really am."

"Does this have anything to do with Jack?"

"No! Fuck you! I would never get upset over a man!" I start bawling even harder.

I sit down next to him on the stoop, and he puts his arm around me and pulls me close as I weep. "I'm really trying to be your friend," he says. "But you make it hard. You stand me up when we had made these plans earlier in the week. Your response to every disagreeable situation is to take some drug. Look at you. Look at what a mess you are. Look at what you're doing to yourself. Clay and I both think you have a drug problem and need professional help." Clay was the music editor of the weekly newspaper, the *Dallas Observer*.

I look at him in shock. Why the hell does everyone always think the problem is drugs?

"David, what I wouldn't give to have a drug problem," I say. "What I wouldn't give for it to be that simple. If I could check into a rehab and come out the other end okay, I'd be thrilled." That was the line I had for everybody, and the sad thing was, like most stereotypes and clichés, it was actually true. I *did* do too many drugs and too much of everything, but there's a qualitative line that I never crossed, that intangible border that separates addicts—people who will need to detox to keep clean—from the rest of us who have our phases and binges, but lack the germ, the tendency toward chemical dependency. My problem always was depression, straight up. The drinking, the drugging, they were mere accessories to the crime. Freshman year in college, that long hot summer in Dallas—those were periods of excess that came and went, never to be repeated. But the vise of depression, no matter what, just wouldn't let go. "It's not drugs," I say to David. "It's just, it's that, it's just that it's all so awful."

When it was 7:00 A.M. and David had finally left after I'd put him through the terrors of listening to all four Grateful Dead albums in tandem, I decided to call my mother.

"Mommy," I whimpered when she picked up the phone. "Mommy, next weekend I'm supposed to get on a plane out of Dallas, and I want to come home. I really want to come home. Everything's wrong. I can't stay here any longer. I miss you. I need to come back."

"Oh, Ellie."

That's all she said at first, and I couldn't tell if she was sympathetic or angry or indifferent or what. I knew that she was mostly amazed that I was awake this early in the morning, and I didn't have the courage to tell her that I hadn't even been to sleep yet, that these days I never got to sleep before this hour.

"Listen, sweetheart," she continued, "I've decided it's really important, wherever you are, that we get you back into therapy, because I can see it's not working too well for you without it."

"I know."

"So somehow, I don't know how, we're going to have to come up with the money."

"Mommy, I don't want you to hate me."

"I don't hate you. Don't be ridiculous. I love you. But sometimes you do terrible things."

"I don't mean to."

"Well, I see that. And I see that you're obviously holding some kind of grudge, I don't know if it's against me or your father or the world, but I feel like if you'd been in therapy earlier, if we'd been able to stick with Dr. Isaac, maybe you wouldn't be this way now. And I feel like that's my fault, that I should really help you get the help you need now so that you'll be all right by the time you get out of Harvard."

"You think it's possible?"

"I don't know," she says. "I hope so."

8

Space, Time, and Motion

✳ ✳ ✳

> She is the rain,
> waits in it for you,
> finds blood spotting her legs
> from the long ride.
> DIANE WAKOSKI
> "Uneasy Rider"

The next semester was going to be great. A recovery period. I would treat Cambridge like a metropolitan mental health retreat, a full course load of Comp Lit, café au lait, and therapy. No boyfriends, no drinking, no drugs, nothing to distract me, pleasantly or otherwise, from my single-minded, stubborn goal of sanity. I would have no life until I knew how to actually live one. Sure, now and again there'd be parties, and of course there would be friends and gossip—friends and gossip are a good thing—but no entanglements. No obsessive-compulsive relationships that are so absorbing that when you're in the middle of one you can't even get through the fashion spreads in *Vogue*, can't even read seven thousand words about Demi Moore in *Vanity Fair*, certainly can't achieve the kind of pellucid concentration it would take to really get into therapy, to work a program, to make the sturdy, rugged steps it would take to lick this depression thing once and for all.

The first thing that needed to be done, once I blew into town and settled into my apartment on Kirkland Street, was to find a decent therapist. Mom would foot the bill because she was totally petrified. She thought nothing less than a medical doctor, preferably one from a top school, like, say, Harvard, would do the trick because she thought I was completely nuts. But my roommate Samantha's father, one of the first lay analysts to be accepted by some important Freudian society in Europe, recommended that I see this psychiatric social worker he had trained. I decided I'd visit all of them, every name that was ever mentioned, whether by Dr. Saltenstahl at U.H.S. or by any of the screwed-up friends I had. I had consultations with so many practitioners that after a while my days were just a long series of door plaques and an alphabet soup mix of titles—Ed.D., M.S.W., Ph.D., A.C.S.W., M.D.—and it struck me as an odd irony that a person as ill equipped as I was to make decisions about almost any important aspect of my life now had to decide who would help correct that condition.

I ultimately chose a psychiatrist who Dr. Saltenstahl recommended to me, a woman who at one time worked at Harvard and now had a private practice in her beautiful colonial home on Mt. Auburn Street. Her name was Diana Sterling, and I liked her because she'd gone to Harvard like me back in the early seventies, was now married to a classmate of hers, and had two kids with the civilized-but-still-trendy names Emma and Matthew who attended a Cambridge private school full of professors' children and Daughters of the American Revolution gone hippie. It seemed to me that she lived an honorable, stable life that made sense to me, unlike so many therapists I'd met who seem to have chosen their profession mainly as a way to exorcise their own demons. I also liked that she wasn't Jewish, that the certain tendencies to overmother or overburden or overcriticize that I had always taken as mere tics of ethnicity would be recognized by Dr. Sterling for the destructive, dysfunctional behaviors that they were. I wanted a therapist who was a role model.

I would see Dr. Sterling in her basement office twice a week. I would tell her about this and that former therapist and this and that bad experience. I would explain my parents, my Jewish education, my New York City upbringing. She would ask a question now and again, but generally the whole atmosphere seemed completely benevolent, almost too placid. I was waiting for the tears, the overwhelming emotions, the catharsis, the drama, the revelations. I was waiting for therapy to bang me over the head and make me say, Ah yes, now I see: *That's* the problem, I should have known all along.

But instead, my life in Cambridge had taken on such a complete calm and uneventfulness that I never had any new incidents to work through, and I felt too unruffled to spend much time dredging up bad memories. I would actually sit on the bus to Dr. Sterling's office trying to think of things to talk about. I felt like a girl heading out for a first date with her dream boy, creating a mental agenda of potential conversation ideas just in case, heaven forbid, there was any kind of lag. I worried that I wasn't entertaining Dr. Sterling enough, I worried that she'd put me on some list of her dull patients that she'd share with her husband late at night, of the ones who couldn't even scare up enough psychodrama in their lives to get themselves through a fifty-minute hour. I worried that my decision to abstain from self-destruction was turning me into a bore. I began to think that in my current state I was too sane for therapy. I started to wonder if maybe my time and money couldn't be better spent sitting around, reading and writing and hoping that the answers would come to me.

And then I got a job working security for the Harvard

Police Department two nights a week. It was a post a lot of students took because they could sit and read during their shift. My hours were from 11:00 at night until 7:00 in the morning, and I was stationed in Adams House, where most of my friends lived, so I would mostly hang out in their rooms downing quart-size cups of coffee from Tommy's Lunch and filling out a log sheet at the end of the shift. The job was good for socializing and getting some reading done, but not seeing the sun two days a week was really hard on me. Even if you woke up at sunrise every morning, Cambridge was a gray, cloudy, lightless place, a city where the days would get shorter and the nights would get long, black, and bitter cold as the winter approached. Missing out on daylight twice a week was very detrimental to my moods since I am extremely photosensitive. Every winter, I would consider going to a tanning salon just to experience some ultraviolet rays. To begin to live in darkness as early as September was almost untenable for me.

Besides the sunshine factor, being up all night two days a week threw my schedule off for the rest of the time, and I started to skip classes and sections when I was too tired to go. The anchoring ports that used to keep my days even were all lost to what seemed like a constant need for sleep. Who had time for lunch, dinner or even a coffee break when you were too zonked to move? To top it off, I decided to live off-campus in one of my moments of folly, though it is pretty rare at Harvard, where the dormitory space is so nice and usually so much cheaper than anything you can find on the local real estate market, so I felt out of touch with the flow of life.

Between my apartment and my job, I was living out of place and out of time.

And I started to get depressed again. One afternoon, after working security the night before, I couldn't remember what day it was, I couldn't figure out what classes I had missed, and I had this twilight-zone sensation in which I almost couldn't figure out if I was in my own bed, my own room, my own head. It was like having a hangover without the alcohol. I felt unsafe and suddenly certain that my apartment was not really my home, that it was just another place I was temporarily tarrying, that like everything else in my life, all I was doing here was passing through. I got out of bed, stumbled down the long corridor toward our bathroom, rinsed my face with water, and felt myself beginning to choke. Next thing I knew, I was on the floor with my head hanging over the toilet bowl, vomiting. I hadn't eaten anything in so long that all that was coming up was bile and other gastric juices, and as soon as I was done my stomach muscles, my diaphragm, and my trachea all felt very sore, as if they'd just done a full Nautilus circuit without me. The taste in my mouth was bitter, but I was too tired to get up and brush my teeth. And then the phone rang.

From the bathroom, I could hear my friend Eben on the answering machine telling me that it was five o'clock, time to leave for the Pink Floyd concert in Hartford that I had, misguidedly, told him I wanted to go to. I ran and picked up the phone and tried explaining to him that I was inexplicably sick, that I'd just thrown up, that I felt as if I might be running a fever.

"That's just from working all night, Liz," he said. "If you get up and go out you'll feel much better."

I knew he was probably right. But somehow I didn't care. I was certain that I couldn't move. "Eben, I can't go to Pink Floyd with you." I started to cry. "Eben." I sniffed. "I'm really sorry. I'll pay for my ticket. I'll pay for yours too. Just please don't give me a hard time, not now. I feel so weak, I don't know what's wrong with me. My head hurts and my body hurts and I'm scared and I don't know why." I kept crying.

"All right, Liz. Whatever."

The next morning, I announced to Dr. Sterling that I felt like I was having a nervous breakdown but I didn't know why. Maybe it was all the darkness and the lack of sleep. Maybe it was the simple fact that the grace period at the beginning of the semester had ended and now reality and routine and depression were kicking in. There were no boys and no booze to blame for this downer, so it was probably just my fate. But whatever it was, it all felt very physical, a psychic ailment that had produced an ague, as if my body were mounting an attack on my mind, and I described the chills, the hot flashes, the nausea, the exhaustion.

"Something is so wrong with me," I groaned. "I'm in so much pain, not just my head but all over, all over, like a bad flu, but one that's definitely emotional even though it's coming out all physical."

I expected Dr. Sterling to think this was all very sudden, that as recently as a few days before I was going on and on about my surprisingly salutary state, but she must have realized that people can crash very suddenly. "All that could be part of the depression," Dr. Sterling said after I described my symptoms. "You've been in therapy about a month, so maybe it's first starting to shake you up now. Maybe you're having your first breakdown. But don't worry: It happens. It's part of the therapeutic process. This is part of how you're going to get better."

And then a few days later I woke up in blood. There was blood on the sheets, blood between the sheets, blood on my nightgown, and I thought I was dying. Actually, I thought I was dead.

And then I felt the plasmatic bits of blood that encrusted

my inner thighs, saw the thick clots of burgundy that traveled down my legs like a run in a pair of stockings. And I thought, Oh no.

I had been vomiting all week before that, but I figured I was just sick as usual. Story of my life. I was so empty that sometimes my body would throw up just to get emptier. But then over the weekend crazy things started to happen. Something in my head hurt so bad that there were hot rushes and hallucinations, and I decided to call my ex-boyfriend Stone and ask him to come over and drink Hungarian red wine with me—so much for no drinking—to take my mind off my mind. And he hugged me for six hours straight because I was scared that if he let go of me I might go jump out the window. My head felt like a plane about to make a crash landing. Or something like that. Actually, it was the levity, the lack of anchoring, that was really starting to frighten me: I was certain that if Stone let go of me I might float up to Mars.

So when I woke up Monday morning surrounded by my own blood, I was sure I was leaving my body for good. I rolled off my futon and pushed myself up and leaned against the wall, creeping slowly down the narrow corridor until I got to the phone. I curled myself around the cradle in a fetal position because the cramps hurt so badly and my lower back felt like it had been clamped with iron tongs and I dialed Stone's number.

I looked behind me and saw a trail of blood, left in dots and splatters on the floor and smears on the wall like a Jackson Pollock painting.

"Stone, I'm dying," I said as soon as he picked up the receiver.

"Again?"

"Stone, I'm dead. I know I said that on Saturday, and I'm sorry to wake you, but there's all this blood and I'm shaking and I'm in pain and I really think I might be dying and maybe I should see a doctor."

"Maybe you have your period."

"Maybe I'm dying, and if you don't come here and take me to the hospital it will be all your fault when I'm dead."

Stone was not one to argue with that kind of skewed logic. It was October 19, 1987. I rode to the infirmary in a taxi wearing only my nightgown with a sweater over it. The blood was everywhere, I was throwing up all over the floor. Other people in the waiting room must have thought of taking their emergencies elsewhere, I was so gross to look at. Meanwhile, the stock market was busy plunging 508 points. I would later note that the market and I both crashed at the same time.

I was lying on the examining table in one of the rooms in the walk-in clinic screaming, "I'm dying! I'm dying!" My stomach felt dreadful sharp pains like ice picks poking at my insides, and finally the nurse said, "Why, sweetheart, you're not dying. If anything, your *baby* is dying."

"My *baby?*" I started to cry. I cried and cried. I thought maybe I would cry an entire nine months. Stone was long gone, so here I was in an antiseptic room full of fluorescent lights with strangers telling me that I'd been pregnant, probably for a couple of months. I hadn't even known I was carrying a baby inside me, and I found out by losing it.

I lose everything.

How on earth could I possibly have been pregnant? Jack, I guessed. There wasn't anyone else. Well, Stone the other night—he thought sex would make me feel more *grounded*— but otherwise nobody. Even Jack, I couldn't remember when or where it happened, or even *that* it happened. But it must have. There was only one Virgin Mary in history, and she didn't have a miscarriage.

"She's a very lucky girl," I heard the doctor saying in the other room as she prepped some equipment to perform a D and C. "Now she won't have to have an abortion."

An abortion?! I couldn't believe the doctor just assumed that's what I'd have done. Maybe I would have, but maybe I would have given the kid up for adoption. Maybe I'd even have been an earthy single mother, carting my baby to day care as I ran off to classes, breast-feeding in the park, making sure that the men I dated liked children. And maybe I *would* have had an abortion. But how could anyone with as little love in her life kill the love growing inside her? I'd sooner kill myself. I'd have sooner killed the doctor standing over me smiling knowingly when she didn't know a thing. In fact, I'd have liked to kill us both. I wanted to burst into tears from all the killing.

Which is what I did. I cried so much that they finally gave me Xanax to calm me down. When that didn't work, two hours later they gave me Valium. When I was still crying late that night, they gave me something like Thorazine and told me I would spend the next few days in the infirmary.

No one would tell her what was wrong with her. She would just lie in her bed, staring at pink walls, taking pink pills that the nurse in white would give her. Between the green pills and the yellow ones. And all these blues.

Actually, I was only in the infirmary overnight. It seemed like days, or ages, because I was doped and disoriented and didn't know where I was or what was happening most of the time, which I guess is the best thing when the alternative is hysteria. The psychologist on duty came in to speak to me, some blood was taken from my arms, a thermometer was stuck in my mouth, and a couple of meals were dispensed, but otherwise my interaction with humans was minimal. At one point, my roommate Samantha came to visit and asked what they were doing for me, and all I could say was, "Giving me pills and letting me sleep."

"This is medieval!" Samantha exclaimed. She went into a rage about how I needed counseling, not drugs. I was too knocked out to explain to her that I was probably too knocked out for anything *but* drugs. It amazed me that Samantha and I hadn't known each other very long—only since we had become roommates through a mutual friend some time in September—and already we had developed this big sister–little sister rapport. Samantha was two years older than I, and had just gotten back from taking a year off from school, during which she lived in London and worked as a bond trader at an investment bank. She was now employed part-time by the same company in Boston, in addition to writing position papers for the Dukakis presidential campaign, promoting the causes of a Colombian dissident named Brooklyn Rivera, flying off to Minnesota on weekends to date one of Walter Mondale's sons, and taking a full load of courses. She even managed to go running a few times a week.

Samantha often told me about how depressed and despondent she'd once been, how she used to cry herself to sleep in her boyfriend's bed in London because she felt so lonely, even lying beside him, and how she'd stand up and walk out in the middle of dinner parties without excusing herself because she needed to burst into tears for no apparent reason. She would tell me these things to assure me that I, too, would get over whatever was ailing me. But it seemed pretty hard to believe I'd ever be as together as Samantha, Samantha who was planning to spend her winter break trekking through Nicaragua and El Salvador on a fact-finding mission for her thesis about postwar diplomacy between Central America and the British government. Samantha couldn't even speak Spanish, but was somehow unfazed by this impediment. Lying in that infirmary bed, the idea of going anywhere with only a thin knowledge of the native tongue, especially a region where dead bodies have been known to turn up in the bathrooms of bus stations, seemed like a task that would require more energy than I would have to expend for the rest of my life. Lying in that infirmary bed, the idea of going to Central America didn't seem impossible just there and then—it seemed impossible forever. I couldn't imagine *ever* getting better.

That's the thing about depression: A human being can survive almost anything, as long as she sees the end in sight. But depression is so insidious, and it compounds daily, that it's impossible to ever see the end. The fog is like a cage without a key.

I was almost happy for a little while after I got out of the infirmary. My other roommate, Alden, brought me a bouquet of fuchsia flowers when she got home that day, and we sat around and laughed about how there I thought I was going crazy, when really it was just a miscarriage. We drank white wine and toasted to the happy future I would have now that I knew what was wrong.

As if I knew.

Suddenly my problems seemed to have a physical cause, and I was more satisfied with somatic explanations than the usual psychic ones. When I told close friends that I'd just had a miscarriage, that I hadn't even known I was pregnant until my body had ejected the fetus, they all seemed to have much more sympathy—even much more retroactive sympathy— for me than when it was all just depression and all so ineffable. As a result, I kept playing up the miscarriage issue, even long after my cramps, my *terrible* cramps, had subsided and I had all but forgotten about it. At first, I was hush-hush about having been pregnant, making the few friends who knew swear to keep it a secret. But after a while I couldn't help myself. I inspired such kindness and pity in people by just mentioning the word *pregnancy*. And when I went on to explain that I hadn't been aware of what had happened to me, that after I'd been knocked up I'd become so alienated from my own body that I hadn't even noticed that I was missing periods until I actually woke up one day soaked in my own blood—when I added in that factor, I could always arouse some feminist outrage.

I had become so good at saying, glibly, *Don't give me a hard time, I've just had a miscarriage*, that I almost forgot that it was the truth. I felt like hell. I was physically drained and emotionally empty, and according to my accounting, I didn't think I'd be able to get away with using the I-was-pregnant-and-didn't-know-it-until excuse for very much longer.

"You don't need an excuse to be depressed," Dr. Sterling told me in one of our sessions. "You just are. You have to stop feeling guilty about it. Feeling guilty is just making you more depressed."

"This is going to sound dumb," I began, far too aware that everything I said was so trite, "but, the thing is, I really don't feel like I have a right to be so miserable. I know we can look back and say my father neglected me, my mother smothered me, I was perpetually in an environment that was incoherent to me, but—" But what? What other excuses do you need? I wasn't feeling gross enough to mention Bergen-Belsen, cancer, cystic fibrosis, and all the other *real* reasons to be sorrowful. "But a lot of people have hard childhoods," I continued, "much harder than mine, and they grow up and get on with it."

"A lot of them don't."

"I don't care about the ones who don't. I think I should be among those who do. I've been so lucky in so many ways, had so many compensations—" It made me sick listening to myself. How many times and to how many therapists had I made this speech? When would I stop wondering what right—what *nerve*—I had to be depressed? Enough with this going on about all my blessings. I was starting to sound like a character in a TV movie with a title like *The Best Little Girl in the World* or *Most Likely to Succeed*. "I don't know. The only good thing about this miscarriage is it's given me a reason to feel lousy."

"So you like tangible reasons?"

"Yes, of course. Doesn't everybody?"

"Well, no, not necessarily."

"That's the reason a suicide try has always appealed to me. I mean, since I've been such a cosmic failure in my numerous attempts to get addicted to drugs and alcohol, the only terrible thing I can see happening would be if I were to overdose or something. Then people would think I was really sick and not just kind of depressed, which is what they think now."

"You've got to stop worrying about what other people think and try to just concentrate on what you feel."

"Oh God," I said, "all I ever do is think about how I feel, and all I ever feel is terrible."

"Well," Dr. Sterling replied with a sigh, before announcing it was time for us to stop, "I guess that's why you're here."

There's something I'm not saying, never even said to Dr. Sterling. Because there are all these things that, as a middle-class, college-educated woman—especially one who is in her early twenties, who has biology and time and future on her side—you're not supposed to feel about getting pregnant. You're never supposed to think, I wanted that baby, or I wish I could have kept it, or anything like that. Pregnancy is just bad luck, a minor inconvenience, something to be dealt with by a simple surgical procedure that doesn't even require hospitalization. There is some pain involved, cramps like having a bad period; and there is some depression involved, but that's just hormones run amok. I've accompanied so many friends to their 8:00 A.M. abortion appointments at St. Acme's Women's Health Center, or whatever the place was called, that it's practically a rite of passage, both to have one and to be the supportive friend who waits while somebody else is having one.

I didn't know I was pregnant, so I never needed to think about having an abortion, but if I had known, I wouldn't have had to think about it either. I would have just done it, no questions asked, no discussions raised. Okay, maybe I would have created a pretense of choice, maybe I would have sat with a counselor or nurse practitioner at U.H.S. and discussed my other options, talked about carrying the pregnancy to term, talked about adoption or single motherhood, but it would have been part of a routine. I would have sat and examined the possibility of not aborting with about as much conviction as a public defender has to give when he is representing a rapist or murderer who he knows is guilty but who has a right to a fair trial anyway. It would have been part of a charade meant to make me believe that when I later marched on Washington in 1989 and again in 1992 demanding a woman's right to choose, I actually believed that idea about choice. There is no choice for a girl like me: There's only abortion.

And if a guy behaves honorably these days, does the right thing when he knocks a girl up, it means he accompanies her to the abortion clinic. Maybe he even pays for half or all of it. Maybe he does his I feel your pain bit. Maybe he says stuff like, It was my child too. But shotgun weddings are now passé. Walking down the aisle is no longer the gentlemanly thing to do. There aren't rules like that any longer. Of course, I know it's better this way. No unwanted babies, no teenage brides and peach-fuzz grooms trapped in marriages that never should have happened. I know it's better.

I know.

No-fault divorce is better too. And still, I can't quite shake this feeling that we live in a world gone wrong, that there are all these feelings you're not supposed to have because there's no reason to anymore. But still they're there, stuck somewhere, a flaw that evolution hasn't managed to eliminate yet, like tonsils or an appendix.

I want so badly to feel bad about getting pregnant, beyond, of course, the surprise and shock. But I can't, don't dare to. Just like I didn't dare tell Jack that I was falling in love with him when I was down in Texas, wanting to be a modern woman who's supposed to be able to handle the casual nature of these kinds of relationships. I'm never supposed to say, to Jack or anyone else, What makes you think I'm so rich that you can steal my heart and it won't mean a thing?

Sometimes I wish I could walk around with a HANDLE WITH CARE *sign stuck to my forehead. Sometimes I wish there were a way to let people know that just because I live in a world without rules, and in a life that is lawless, doesn't mean that it doesn't hurt so bad the morning after. Sometimes I think that I was forced to withdraw into depression because it was the only rightful protest I could throw in the face of a world that said it was all right for people to come and go as they please, that there were simply no real obligations left. Certainly deceit and treachery in both romantic and political relationships is nothing new, but at one time, it was bad, callous, and cold to hurt somebody. Now it's just the way things go, part of the growth process. Really nothing is surprising. My father had a child that he didn't have too much trouble walking away from; it seems only natural that so many of us have pregnancies that we can abandon even more easily. After a while, meaning and implication detach themselves from everything. If one can be a father and assume no obligations, it follows that one can be a boyfriend and do nothing at all. Pretty soon you can add friend, acquaintance, coworker, and just about anyone else to the long list of people who seem to be part of your life, though there is no code of conduct that they must adhere to. Pretty soon, it seems unreasonable to be bothered or outraged by much of anything because, well, what did you expect? In a world where the core social unit—the family—is so dispensable, how much can anything else mean?*

There is a chill as I think of the way being deprived of normal feelings has the paradoxical effect of turning me into an emotional wreck. As Russian writer Aleksandr Kuprin put it: "Do you understand, gentlemen, that all the horror is in just this: that there is no horror!"

It was during a play on the following Friday night when I really cracked. It was a Sam Shepard play. Ruby had produced it. It must have been four hours long. It was one of Shepard's more obscure works, the kind repertory companies dragged out once the possibilities of *Fool for Love* and *True West* had been exhausted. Not that it would have taken much to upset me that night, as I'd just gotten out of the infirmary a few days before and my uteral lining was still hemorrhaging something awful and I was starting to think that maybe a Red Cross blood bank should open a chapter between my legs. Given the circumstances, all it took was one uncomfortable exchange with Ruby before the show started and I was bonkers.

About that time, Ruby had just started dating Gunnar, this guy in my semiotics class who looked like Cary Grant with long hair. It seems she still hadn't recovered from the time I attempted to steal her boyfriend from her freshman year, and she was convinced that I was trying to seduce Gunnar in the middle of lectures about Charles Peirce's linguistics and Lévi-Strauss's anthropology and the Russian formalists and the Frankfurt School and how it all related to a new way of reading Grimm's fairy tales. With all this intellectual mumbo jumbo going on, I could hardly have paid attention to Gunnar if I'd wanted to. And besides, I already had a crush on this other guy who was the whole reason I was taking this ridiculous class in the first place.

More to the point, I was such a basket case, had just gone through this physically punishing mess, that the last thing on my mind was trying to create a new catastrophe by taking off with Ruby's new boyfriend. But when Ruby, Gunnar, and I stood around the theater lobby before the show, and I reached out my hand to straighten Gunnar's crooked tie—a tie he was wearing in her honor since it was her opening night—Ruby considered this some sort of violation. I wasn't supposed to be touching her man, so she got all huffy and refused to talk to me for the rest of the evening. I apologized over and over again, followed her around the theater as she set brownies and large bottles of wine on tables for the after-show party, offered to carry some trays, but Ruby wouldn't speak to me except to say, "*You* can't be trusted."

"Ruby, please, I'm sorry," I kept saying. "Whatever I did, I'm sorry. Please don't be angry at me. I'm not doing very well right now. I need my friends to be nice. I need you."

After the show, Gunnar's roommate Timothy was talking to me for reasons that I couldn't understand. I mean, there I was, losing a pint of blood an hour, one of my best friends was refusing to acknowledge me, so it seemed unbelievable that anyone would want to be nice. Timothy was trying to engage me in some sort of discussion of the play's dominant motifs, but all I wanted to talk about was how mean Ruby was being. I didn't know why I was having this conversation with him. I barely knew him, and heaven knows this was no way to get a guy interested. You were supposed to be peppy and bright for boys, no matter how bad you felt inside. At least that's what Mother always told me. *Don't let him see how crazy you are,* she'd say. *No one wants anyone who's down like you.* But all Timothy was to me that night was all anyone ever was to me at that point: a new person to sob to. Someone who hadn't yet heard the spiel, someone for whom my depression, my problems real and imaginary, and everything about me were not just a matter of there-she-goes-again.

"Life is so horrible," I said, as Timothy and I sat down at an outdoor café, taking in a final bit of Indian summer before the deep freeze. "Life is awful, Ruby treats me horribly, I just want to die."

"No you don't," he said. What was he supposed to say? We'd known each other only twenty minutes. Well, no time for small talk these days.

"Really I do," I insisted. "I have no reason to lie to you. I hardly know you. I had a miscarriage the other day, it all seems like shit to me, and now Ruby, who's supposed to be one of my best friends, won't talk to me. These seem like, taken together, adequate reasons for suicide."

When he didn't answer me, I realized suddenly that I knew Timothy, that he'd dated Hadley, one of my freshman-year neighbors, a girl who had been doing her first year over again because during her initial try at Harvard she'd tried to kill herself twice and wound up in McLean for a couple of months. Timothy was the one who she, still in a bit of a stupor a year later, would always refer to as the great love of her life.

"God, it just occurred to me." I asked, "You're not the Timothy that Hadley always talked about?"

"I'm the one."

And so I prattled a bit about how I'd heard so much about him, and he explained to me that Hadley greatly exaggerated the extent of their relationship in her own mind, mainly because he was really nice to her while she was losing it.

"You know, when Hadley was in McLean, I was the only one who visited her there," he said.

"Oh."

"I know you don't really want to kill yourself. You just

want to end up at some hospital where you can take a break for a while."

"Maybe."

"Not maybe," he said, with force. "*Definitely.* I know what you're thinking." He was so adamant in that been-there-done-that way that I couldn't argue with him. "Well, I used to go visit Hadley there and that's why I can tell you that it's really horrible. When you get committed, it's not like they send you to some farm in the mountains where you take long walks in the country and quietly reflect. It's not all art therapy either. Mostly you just lie in your horrible bed and do nothing. The doctors check up on you from time to time and you go to group with people who are so much further gone than you are that you can't figure out what you're doing with them. Plus hospitals are sterile, really white, really light blue and light pink. The TVs hang from the ceiling. The food is terrible. If you can get better out here, I don't know why you'd want to go in there."

"Maybe I don't think I can." I found myself suddenly annoyed that Timothy was trying to tell me what to do. Maybe I like bad food and sterile decor and TVs hanging from the ceiling. Besides, maybe I really did want to die. How would he know?

"Timothy, listen, this has been fun and enlightening, but I've got to run," I said. "I've got to write some Space, Time, and Motion papers." This was true enough. I did have a lot of catching up to do in a physics class that I'd joined two weeks late. I smiled as if to say, What a nerd I am, doing homework on a Friday night.

"Do you really think you're in any condition for that?"

"Sure. Work always makes me feel better." That was true too. "*Arbeit macht frei,*" I added, realizing that Timothy wasn't Jewish and probably wouldn't get my morbid reference to Auschwitz.

"I'm not going to let you go home alone if you're talking about suicide."

"No, I mean it. I really do feel better about myself when I'm being productive. I mean, my feeling is that when your friends and everything let you down, there's always worth-while shit to be done that you've been putting off anyway, so I think I'll go home and do that."

"Elizabeth," Timothy said, "it's after one. Why don't you just go home and sleep?"

"Oh, I can't. Can't do anything until I write my papers. I can always sleep tomorrow."

"I think you need sleep now. I think sleep would make you feel better."

I gathered my belongings and headed across Harvard Yard toward my apartment. Timothy followed along. "Look, Timothy, I'm going home, I'm doing what I need to do, and I'm gonna be fine." I smiled. "And if for some strange reason I'm dead by tomorrow morning, be sure to tell Ruby that I'll consider forgiving her in the hereafter."

"I'm not letting you go back there—" he began to say, but by that time I'd already made a run for it, sprinting across the Yard and speeding down Kirkland Street. At some point, I guess Timothy must have decided I was out of his hands because I made it home alone.

When I get home, Alden tries to involve me in some late-night chatter, begins to tell me about some dance performance she went to, as if I might care. Clearly, Alden has no idea that all that matters is Space, Time, and Motion, a class that I have no clue about, though I am still somehow convinced that it can redeem my whole life. I have to write some papers, and everything will be fine.

I walk, surefooted, straight toward my bedroom, but Alden hears that I'm beginning to cry and she follows me. I fall onto my floor, my bag and coat and body all in a pile like a heap of junk, a weeping heap of junk. Alden watches, not sure what to do. Still crying, I walk toward my desk, and pick up a Space, Time, and Motion source book, carry it to my bed, and open it up as if I were going to read it.

"Listen, Elizabeth," Alden suggests, coming closer, "I think you need to sleep and I think you need to calm down. Why don't you save your work for tomorrow."

"If I can get through this," I mumble, "if I can read this Darwin, I'll be all right. If I can do what I need to do, I'll be fine."

"Elizabeth, this is crazy."

"And then, if I die any time soon, at least they'll be able to say that I led a productive life and did all my work on time. I may be dead, but I'll be up to date in Space, Time, and Motion."

I lean back on my bed, put the book against my bent knees, and try to read even though my eyes are blurry from tears. Alden walks over and pulls the book away. "Why won't you tell me what's wrong?"

"Because it doesn't matter anymore. Nothing matters anymore."

"Jesus, Elizabeth, Samantha's asleep, I don't know what to do here. What do you want me to do? I'm worried about you."

"I'll be fine," I scream. "I'll be fine if you'll just let me write my Space, Time, and Motion papers!"

She leaves my room and heads for the phone. She calls the emergency room of the infirmary and talks to the psychiatrist on duty. She tells her about my miscarriage, about how unhappy I've been, about how I'm threatening suicide. Finally, Alden pulls me out of my room and puts me on the phone. I'm still crying.

"What's the matter?" the doctor asks.

"Nothing," I say. "I just have work to do."

"Okay, I understand that, but it's late at night and it sounds like what you really need is some sleep."

"Goddamnit!" I scream. "Everyone is so fucking fixated on this sleep thing. I'm either writing my papers or I'm killing myself. Got it?"

"Maybe you should come back to Stillman if that's how you feel," she suggests. "A hospital environment might help you."

"But I can't." This is getting very frustrating, I think. "I CAN'T GO TO STILLMAN BECAUSE I HAVE TO WRITE MY SPACE, TIME, AND MOTION PAPERS, OR I'M GOING TO GET REALLY DERAILED. WHY DOESN'T ANYBODY UNDERSTAND THAT EVERYTHING WILL BE FINE IF I CAN JUST READ DAR-WIN IN PEACE?"

The doctor obviously doesn't understand this because she says that she is sending a couple of orderlies to get me and deliver me to the infirmary tonight. She says something about not wanting to leave me to my own devices right now. I'm crying as I listen and I cry even more when I see Alden stand-ing over me nervously, wanting to make sure that I really will be entrusted into safe hands. The doctor says she will give me time to pack a bag and take what I need and that a car will be outside in ten minutes.

"Okay?" she asks before hanging up. "So I'll see you over at Stillman shortly."

"All right, but I'm bringing my work," I say. "I have to finish my Space, Time, and Motion papers, or it'll all be over."

"That's fine," the doctor says, with just the right amount of condescension. "Bring whatever you want."

There's not a lot to do at Stillman besides read and watch TV. Doctors come in every few hours and interview me, ask me what's wrong and how I plan to make it right. And I say I don't know, because I don't. They administer pills, mostly Dalmane, so I can sleep and stop talking about Space, Time, and Motion and all my overdue papers. And even I have to admit that in this insulated room, things do seem okay. Timothy was wrong. Inside here it is sterile, it is drab, the light is artificial and too bright, but at least no one can touch me.

9

Down Deep

✳ ✳ ✳

God have mercy on the man
Who doubts what he's sure of.
BRUCE SPRINGSTEEN
"Brilliant Disguise"

I don't know if depressives are drawn to places with that certain funereal ambience or if, in all their contagion, they make them that way. I know only that for my entire junior year of college, I slept under a six-foot-square poster emblazoned with the words LOVE WILL TEAR US APART, and then I wondered why nothing good ever happened in that bed.

But it wasn't just my bedroom. It was the whole apartment. It felt sickly, shady. I wouldn't be surprised to learn that it's been turned into a crack house or a shooting gallery since I moved out. Or better still, a halfway house for recovering vampires. The place was as dark at noon as it was at midnight. It was the perfect site for a nervous breakdown. My apartment in Texas, with all its airy, sunny decorator touches, may have been a place for some pretty nasty precursors to disaster, but it took the haunted house I settled into in Cambridge to finish off the job.

Since I barely left my bed after my miscarriage, except

to roam the streets of Cambridge late at night, I lived my life, quite literally, in the dark. While our living room, with its southern exposure, was full of sun, no one ever spent any time in there because, ever since we'd decided to hide the ugly brown plaid couches under white cotton sheets, it looked like we were holding a wake. The rest of the house and all of the bedrooms that pimpled off the long corridor in our railroad flat faced a courtyard to the north. And all of us, either because we were depressed or tired or had schoolwork, cocooned ourselves in our dark but, paradoxically, vast rooms, lost in our troglodyte existence. The whole apartment seemed infected with some kind of craziness: Alden with her Zen Buddhism, meditating ten hours a day; and Samantha with her type A, overachiever schedule, afraid that if she slowed down, she'd turn into someone like me.

We had a fourth roommate, Sindhi, a Pakistani woman who went out with my friend Paul. When she finally decided that she could just shack up with him, that her parents in Karachi would never be the wiser, we replaced her with a series of roommates, all of whom dropped out of school or dropped out of life as soon as they moved in with us. Jean-Baptiste, a French student of artificial intelligence at M.I.T., decided to return to Paris and learn to play the oboe within two months of living with us. Inigo, a British graduate student of American history at Harvard, decided to return to his family's farm in Shropshire and take up sheepherding within a month of settling in. W.B., a recent Harvard graduate, stayed with us for many months, and even though we all loved him to death, his mental health deteriorated during his tenure as our roommate. One day he was an editor at *Sail* magazine, the next day a bike messenger, the next day he was applying to law school, the next he was moving to L.A. to write screenplays. Both he and I began to suspect that this was the

apartment from hell, that a miasma of depression and con-
fusion had infiltrated the walls.

In fact, when Alden left to go back to school at Barnard
in New York because she was just a visiting student at Harvard, my friend Veronica moved into Alden's old room and
promptly got depressed. Veronica was taking her second semester senior year off because she couldn't—simply *could
not*—write her thesis. Every time she sat at her Macintosh to
work, she got physically ill and claustrophobic and paralyzed,
which is why she moved in with us. Of course, after only a
few weeks on Kirkland Street, with the nasty breakup with
her boyfriend and a sudden inability to get out of bed before
four in the afternoon, the least of Veronica's problems was
her thesis. Needless to say, except for Samantha, who was a
Woman with a Purpose, which is in itself kind of fucked up,
everyone in the apartment was certifiable.

So many people had lived in this four-bedroom apartment over the years that it reeked of adolescence relived again
and again. Patches of acne medicine permanently encrusted
the bathroom sink, and the mirrored cabinet was full of left-
over Bactrim prescriptions and the like, remnants of urinary
tract infections gone by. The apartment was cheap and big,
with a Mop & Glo-ad type of kitchen, but no one ever
seemed to stay in it for more than a year, knowing somehow
that they were lucky to get out alive.

*I become one of those people who walks alone in the dark at night
while others sleep or watch* Mary Tyler Moore *reruns or pull all-
nighters to finish up some paper that's due first thing tomorrow. I
always carry lots of stuff with me wherever I roam, always weighted
down with books, with cassettes, with pens and paper, just in case I
get the urge to sit down somewhere, and oh, I don't know, read
something or write my masterpiece. I want all my important posses-
sions, my worldly goods, with me at all times. I want to hold what*

little sense of home I have left with me always. I feel so heavy all the time, so burdened. This must be a little bit like what it's like to be a bag lady, to drag your feet here, there, and everywhere, nowhere at all.

It is October, too chilly for this kind of wandering. But I must move, must get farther and farther away from this fire that's going to burn all of me down. It is cold outside, but I'm crazy from the heat.

I wake up the afternoon after Halloween to darkness as usual, and I can't get out of bed. It is a Sunday, and Sundays are so drab, nothing to do but catch up on schoolwork and feel hung over and consume aspirin. The only thing good about Sundays when I was living on campus were the Cocoa Krispies for brunch, a supreme treat for someone who grew up on sugar-free Total and granola. But now, I tell myself as I lie on my futon on the floor of my room, I live off campus and there is nothing to eat in this whole apartment because going to the supermarket is too much of an effort for me because I have nothing else to do, and too much of an effort for Samantha because she has too much else to do.

Okay, I think, lying in my bed, Let's face it, girl, you live in fucking anomie here. Of course you're going crazy, Elizabeth. People tend to go crazy when they don't even have a container of milk in the refrigerator.

So I push myself up from bed as if I were a tape ejecting from a player. As I pad into the kitchen to make myself some tea, I decide to call my mother. What I need, I think, is to do something *real* normal. Something that's normal and that gives me a sense of connectedness with the world. Because right now I feel a bit like a tree cut from the ground on its way to the lumberyard for further cutting. And the thing about my mom is that she's totally nuts, but she's very normal. She pays taxes, she works for a living, she boils water without burning the pot. She's so far from my present surroundings that I think calling her will somehow transport me to a saner place. We used to talk every day almost, but we haven't lately because there's too much I don't want to tell her and too much she doesn't want to know. Our silence is a cooperative venture, although we still chat about nothing every few days. Maybe it's time we had a serious conversation.

As soon as she picks up the phone, she starts yelling about something. Partly it's that she called a few days ago and I haven't gotten back to her until now, partly it's that she's just received a pharmacy bill from Harvard and she wants to know what all this medicine is about, partly she yells because that is what she does. I come from a family of screamers. If they are trying to express any emotion or idea beyond pass the salt, it comes in shrieks. So my mom is the opposite of composure, and I am calling her with the sole hope that her maternal stability will seep through the fiber-optic lines.

I almost say to her, *Mommy, I'm coming to you with a need, and you're going to have to fill it, or at least fake it for a while, because I need you to be a motherly mother who believes I can do no wrong right now.* And you know, I feel so desperate that I would say it if I thought it would work.

But it won't. There have been countless times when she's been hysterical and I've begged her to calm down because she is the only adult in my life I can trust and when she gets crazy I feel as if the bottom is slipping and sliding out from under me, but this doesn't stop her. She does not look at me with comprehension or recognition, as if what I'm saying makes enough sense for her to stop screaming. She never steps back and sees that her behavior is inappropriate or disproportionate, or, worst of all, not productive. She keeps screaming. And I sit around plotting and planning, wondering what I would have to do to shut off the noise, what state of desperation would I have to achieve before she'd realize that the way she's carrying on is killing me.

Rest assured, it's not going to happen on this dreary Sunday afternoon. I get off the phone with my mother, worse for the wear, and wonder what's left.

I dialed Rafe's number, something I'd been meaning to do for four years, after I hung up with my mother.

I didn't know what I was expecting—I'd met him only once, during my junior year of high school when I was looking at colleges and visited Brown—but salvation would have done the trick. Rafe was a friend of a friend, we'd been introduced only because his parents were suing each other over the same issues mine were, he didn't talk to his dad either, and our mutual friend thought we might enjoy exchanging notes from divorce court. I think we had, but that was four years ago.

I didn't know how to tell him that it was up to him to save my life now.

When he answered the phone, I almost remembered the voice. "Hello? Is this Rafe?"

"It is."

"Hi, Rafe, my name is Elizabeth, and I'm a friend of Jim Witz's. We met a few years ago when I came to Brown for a visit because I was choosing schools."

"Uh-huh." No sign of recognition.

"Well, anyway, at the time Jim introduced us, I think mainly because I had all these problems with my father and you had similar ones with yours . . ." I could tell by his lack of responsiveness, his failure to sigh or groan or do anything to suggest he knew what I meant, that he'd completely forgotten the encounter. "Anyway, you probably don't remember, it was just one evening so long ago," I added to keep from embarrassing myself.

"Maybe if you told me what you look like, I'd remember," he suggested.

"Well, you know, the truth is I came up there the first week of your freshman year so probably it's all a big haze to you now." Just answer the question, Elizabeth. "But since you ask, I have very long light brown hair and dark eyes, and I wear black a lot, which probably makes me sound like every other girl you know."

"Yeah, well, that pretty much covers almost everyone around here."

"Look, the real reason I called"—what *was* the real reason I called?—"is that, um, I'm trying to track Jim down and I thought you might know where he is now that he graduated."

"No idea." So much for that pretext.

"Okay, well, then I guess I won't bother you with this anymore."

"Hey, wait a minute," he said, finally showing some enthusiasm. "You can't hang up. You still haven't told me what's happened to you since I met you a few years ago."

"But you don't remember anyway."

"Well, I do vaguely."

!!!!!!!!!!

"Well, let's see, I'm a junior at Harvard now, I'm studying Comparative Literature, I write a lot, other than that I think it's pretty safe to say that nothing eventful has happened to me in the last few years." A miscarriage, a prelude to a nervous breakdown, nothing eventful. "And I still don't talk to my father, though it's not for lack of trying."

For some reason, we talked about what bands and authors we liked, and then he started telling me about his plans to return to Minneapolis, his hometown, after graduation, to try to make it as an actor. He told me that he just finished starring in a run of an updated version of Molière's *Tartuffe*. He told me that he wished I could have seen it, it was great. And I thought to myself, as women do, Why does he wish I could see it? Is it because as an actor he wishes everyone could see his performances? Or is it *me* he wants there?

In the meantime, I told him that I was really sorry that he couldn't tell me where to find Jim, but now I had to go. "But good luck with everything," I said. "I hope it all works out for you."

"Wait a minute," he said. "Wait, wait. Just let me get your number in case I'm ever in Boston."

"Why would you want that?"

"Well, so I can call you when I'm up there. Maybe we can meet again or something."

"Oh, I see." So cool. Elizabeth, you have never been so cool in your life. "I suppose that would be fine."

"I might even be there really soon. A good friend of mine is from Cambridge," he says. "And my roommate's from Arlington."

"Oh, how nice," I say. How nice. "Well, give a call then."

Two days later, on Tuesday night, I was back on the phone with Rafe.

"Hi, it's me again," I said when he picked up, as if we were already familiar. "Listen, this may sound strange, but I was thinking, um . . ." Um. "Could I come visit you this weekend? I really need to get away from here, and I don't really have anywhere else to go but home, which isn't—"

He cut me off with laughter. "The funny thing is," he said, "for the last couple of days, I've been trying to figure out ways I could get up to Boston so I could see you."

By 4:00 A.M. on Friday night, we had been to a play, we had been to a couple of parties, and we had been back at Rafe's house a couple of hours, and he still hadn't kissed me. And I didn't know what to do.

Rafe's apartment was quite nice, the kind of place that

the Brown housing office awards you with as a senior. He shared it with two roommates, and a friend who got thrown out of a fraternity occupied the attic space. But even at that very late hour, nobody was home except Rafe and me. We sat and talked on the day bed in the living room. I was half scared that he was actually going to suggest that I sleep there since he was very sensitive about the fact that I'd recently been through this gynecological nightmare, and he was probably the kind of guy who would think that separate beds was the right thing to do.

I was petrified that this really was going to be just a weekend away, some time to regroup and return to Harvard a bit refreshed. I was so scared that Rafe was not going to be my salvation after all, and I couldn't deal with that. He had to be.

He had to be.

And just when I was feeling completely ominous, thinking that I could have spent this weekend doing, well, frankly, my Space, Time, and Motion papers instead of hanging out with a guy who wants only to be caring and compassionate and politically correct; just when I was remembering there were so many things I should have been doing, that I am not here for anything other than salvation; just then, when I could stand it no longer, Rafe finally kissed me.

Saved.

I see him every weekend. Sometimes that means from Friday to Sunday, but more and more often it means from Thursday to Monday. When we are together, all we are is together. No work gets done, no play rehearsals, no cleaning, not much cooking. The three days that I am in Cambridge, I struggle to get through what I have to, to do my reading, to write my papers, to wash my laundry, to go to my new job at Lamont Library, even to attend classes. But it is so hard to care about anything or anybody at Harvard. I live in complete darkness, hoping each day that Rafe will call me or planning to call him.

Every so often, I look around at my apartment. I see that all the posters that I so carefully chose and taped to the living room walls in September are falling as the cold freezes the stickiness out of the tape. I know they need reinforcing, but I let them slip onto the rug and onto the sofas and onto the wing chairs. There are several bags of garbage accumulating in the kitchen, and I know that if someone doesn't do something about it we are going to have rats living with us. I know this but somehow can't seem to remember to pick up one of the bags on my way out in the morning. Can't remember anything except *Where's Rafe?*

I became rambunctious with tears every time I left Rafe. I cried on the bus from Providence to Boston. I cried on the T from Boston to Cambridge. I cried as I walked from Harvard Square to my apartment. I cried when I arrived home and found that my roommates had all gone to sleep and there was no one to cry to. I kept crying on and off for hours. I'd sit at my word processor and type my Space, Time, and Motion papers for the week, since this was the only class I was still bothering to keep up with, and I cried some more between thoughts on Kant and a priori knowledge, or Hopi dialects and the space-time continuum, or non-Euclidean geometry and light rays.

I'd wake up in the morning still crying and I'd start to wonder if it was possible that I'd been crying in my sleep all night long. The only way I could doze off on nights like that was by sneaking one of Alden's Halcion pills out of the bottle she kept in her desk drawer. Inevitably, as soon as I'd wake up in the morning, with that sudden post-Halcion jolt, I'd run for the telephone. I'd call Rafe to tell him that I couldn't stop crying, that I didn't know why, even though he was never sure what to do or say.

I am crying about the elusive nature of love, the impossibility of ever having someone so completely that he can fill up the hole, the gaping hole that for me right now is full of depression. I understand why people sometimes want to kill their lovers, eat their lovers, inhale the ashes of their dead lovers. I understand that this is the only way to possess another person with the kind of desperate longing that I have to take Rafe inside of me.

After a while, it got so that even when I was with Rafe it was not enough. He was always too far away. Even when we were having sex, even when he was as deep inside of me as a living person could be, he was still so far away, he was still on Mars, on Jupiter, on Venus, as far as I was concerned.

I spent a lot of my time away from Rafe crying, and I spent most of my time with him doing the same. When I explained this to Dr. Sterling, when I told her that Rafe was the best boyfriend I had ever had, that as far as I could tell he was completely devoted, and still I cried and cried and cried, she was not sure what was wrong.

"I think the closeness that you're able to experience when you're with Rafe is something you've been deprived of and something you've needed for so long that it's causing you to go to these extremes of emotion every time you feel him slipping away," Dr. Sterling suggested. "I just think the contrast between being with him and being away from him is too much for you to handle."

"But a lot of the times I get all upset I *am* with him," I answered. "It seems like no amount of reassurance from him can convince me that he's really mine."

"There must be a reason you feel this way," Dr. Sterling

said. "You're not a completely irrational being. Something he does must be tipping you off."

I felt the flood packing water behind my eyes. Hot water and hot blood and hot salt. I felt the tears welling up as I started to talk about everything I did to be with Rafe and the way he made no effort to be with me, taking it for granted that I would arrive, gift-wrapped, with a big bow tied around my neck, each and every weekend like I was put on earth just to love and serve him. I knew I had created this situation, but I still hated him for letting me be this way. Hated him for not doing more. Hated him for never coming to see me in Cambridge, for always begging off because he had a play to attend or a paper to write. Hated him because he made me drop everything without even asking me to.

"It's just that, all his words, all that he says about loving me so much, they all don't seem to matter when I feel like this relationship would not be happening at all if it weren't for my efforts," I cried.

"What does this remind you of?"

"My father, of course." Why did she even ask? Did she think I was new to therapy? Did she think I couldn't make these connections on my own? "Of course it's like my dad who never did anything, who never visited, who never called, who never bought me presents, who never invited me to see him, but would still swear to me on the rare occasions that he turned up that he really did love me. Rafe keeps telling me he loves me, but for all I know it's just words."

"I think you need to tell him that," Dr. Sterling suggested. "I think it's very important for you that he come to Cambridge sometime soon, and I think you need to let him know that."

"Do you think he really loves me?"

"I don't know," she answered, beginning to look impatient because she hated my habit of asking her to be omniscient about the feelings of people she'd never met. She sighed. "All I know is that he says he does, and he has no reason to lie."

"You're going to leave me, aren't you?" I asked accusingly when Rafe finally came to Cambridge and all I could do all weekend was cry. "You've had enough of me, haven't you? You're probably so tired of all this crying and all these moods, and I've got to tell you, so am I. So am I. Sometimes it seems like my mind has a mind of its own, like I just get hysterical, like it's something I can't control at all. And I don't know what to do, and I feel so sorry for you because you don't know what to do either. And I'm sure you're going to leave me." More tears.

"Why don't you let me decide about that," he said as he handed me a plate. He'd taken it upon himself to cook some dinner for me—pasta with Bolognese sauce, nothing too complicated, he claimed—because he thought it wouldn't be bad if, just once, I had a home-cooked meal in my apartment. "First of all, I think what you really need to do to feel better is to eat something, because you haven't had a bite since I got here; and second of all, I think I can handle you pretty well. I'm completely sturdy. I'm just worried about you. I'm worried that you can't handle yourself. I love you, Elizabeth, I really do. I love you even when you get like this. But it just scares me. It scares me for your sake. Whatever negative effect you're having on the people who love you, I'm sure it's not half as bad, I'm sure it's not a small percentage as bad, as what you're doing to yourself. You're going to drive yourself crazy."

"I know."

"What does your therapist say?"

"Oh, you know." You know, all the usual stuff therapists say to their crazy patients, all the usual things about mothers and fathers and early childhood trauma. "I don't really want to talk about that right now. I just, I don't have the energy." I sighed. I was exhausted. I sat up and reached for the plate he'd brought for me and started twisting strands of spaghetti around my fork. "I want to make sure that you're not totally sick of me."

"Elizabeth, for God's sake, I said I'm not." He inhaled dramatically and shook his head. "I love you. I don't know how I can convince you of that. And you know, up until this weekend, I think that maybe things could have gone either way, they could have maybe worked out, they could have just fizzled. But now, tonight, I realized with you getting so upset that I am completely here for you. That we're in this together. Whatever else is bothering you, I don't want you to be worried about me. I realized that this is really serious and important and I never want to leave you, no matter what."

"Really?"

"Yes."

"Really?"

"Yes."

We try, we struggle, all the time to find words to express our love. The quality, the quantity, certain that no two people have experienced it before in the history of creation. Perhaps Catherine and Heathcliff, perhaps Romeo and Juliet, maybe Tristan and Isolde, maybe Hero and Leander, but these are just characters, make-believe. We have known each other forever, since before conception even. We remember playing together in a playpen, crossing paths at F.A.O. Schwarz. We remember meeting in front of the Holy Temple in the days before Christ, we remember greeting each other at the Forum, at the Parthenon, on passing ships as Christopher Columbus sailed to America. We have survived a pogrom together, we have died in Dachau together, we have been lynched by the Ku Klux Klan together. There has been cancer, polio, the bubonic plague, consumption, morphine addiction. We have had children together, we have been children together, we were in the womb together. Our history is so deep and wide and long, we have known each other a million years. And we don't know how to express this kind of love, this kind of feeling.

I get paralyzed sometimes. One day, we are in the shower and I want to say to him, I could be submerged in sixty feet of water right now, never drowning, never even fearing drowning, knowing I would always be safe with you here, knowing that it would be okay to die as long as you are here. I want to say this but don't.

Rafe tells me we won't see each other at all during his four weeks of winter vacation. He says he needs to look after his deranged dowager mother and his eleven-year-old sister, who is going through something awful, some other version of crazy in the head, and might need medical attention.

And I think, Why are so many people Rafe is close to going crazy?

And I think, I don't care about his mother and sister or anyone else in Minneapolis or anywhere else on earth. I know only that there's me and that I won't last a month without Rafe.

I cry so hard and so much after Rafe tells me this, I cry all weekend long without surcease. And I keep screaming, You're going away and you're not coming back! You're going away and you're not coming back!

And he just shakes his head and holds me. He says, Four weeks isn't that long.

And I cry even harder after he says that because I see that he has no idea how long and hard and palpable time is for me, that even four minutes of feeling the way I do right now is too long.

★   ★   ★

When I first got home for vacation, I had dinner with my mother and talked to her about school, about Rafe, about ordinary things, but it was clear to me by late that night that there was no way—*no way*—I was going to survive without him. This heavy sense of not-okayness suddenly leapt on me after dinner, and I didn't know what to do. Because the awful feeling was all over me, I was like a farm covered in locusts, being destroyed. I went out for coffee late at night with my friend Dinah. In some little dive on Amsterdam Avenue, all I did was talk about Rafe and how painful it was to be without him.

Dinah and I had been friends since we were both four, since we met during rest period in kindergarten, and she'd told me her father was a magician and I'd told her my dad was a jeweler-astronaut. She would fill empty 7UP bottles with water and tell me it was a magic potion, and I would promise to bring her an emerald necklace or a piece of the moon next time I saw my dad. We were best friends after that, all through elementary school and all through high school. Even when we went off to different colleges, we were still in constant contact. She knew me better than anyone practically, she'd seen me through my earlier bouts with depression, so she knew the signs. Listening to me talk about Rafe, Dinah looked distressed.

"But, Elizabeth," Dinah said, employing a logic that was cruelly alien to me. "Elizabeth, you're going to see Rafe in a few weeks. People get separated from each other all the time, and then they come back together."

"I know. I just don't think I can bear it."

I spoke of the intolerable pain, though even I could see that I should have been happy to be so in love with somebody for the first time since high school. But I couldn't be. I kept imagining the end, the despair I would suffer when it came, and it made any happiness I had in the present seem not merely ephemeral, but doomed. Because the happier I allowed myself to be now, the more miserable I would be later.

I was like an addict being deprived of my drug of choice. As I sat there without Rafe, desperate for a fix of him, I was certain that heroin withdrawal was not so much different because I ached for him and cried for him and shook for him and got down on my knees and threw up from missing him, as if I were in detox.

I convinced myself that he was lost on the planet or lost in the solar system and that I would never find him. I wouldn't be able to reach him by phone, he'd become inaccessible and I would lose him. I would have to contact the F.B.I., whose agents would be unable to locate him. I imagined living out a fate like that of Horacio Oliveira in Julio Cortázar's novel *Hopscotch*. I thought pitifully of the man who must spend the rest of his days searching for his long lost La Maga, his lover, who has disappeared in Montevideo or into some more disheveled part of Uruguay, a country where the missing probably outnumber the found, a country where you can lose somebody for good, a country that lends itself very well to the vagaries and paranoias of fiction because life and death is everywhere in Latin America.

I explained my fears to Dinah, my conviction that Rafe would fade away or fall into a black hole. And she just said things like, This is crazy, this is crazy, and I had to agree with her. But I couldn't stop it. I couldn't.

There was nothing to my days except roaming the streets of the Upper West Side and thinking about Rafe. I tried to do other things. I meant to see *Fatal Attraction*, but I couldn't get it together to go to the movie theater, knowing that once I was there I'd have to stand in line and it could feel like forever. Dinah took me to a Paul Klee exhibit at the Museum of Modern Art, but I couldn't concentrate on all the abstraction. I had schoolwork to do, but I couldn't do it. I had to write a semiotics paper on motorcycle culture and biker conventions, but every time I picked up *Easy Rider* magazine, it seemed like a herculean effort just to turn the page. I'd fall asleep in the bathtub and lie awake all night in bed. I couldn't even wash my face in the morning, my hands were too tired.

I listened to the new Marianne Faithfull album, *Strange Weather*. It really should have been subtitled "Music to Slit Your Wrists To." I cried when I listened. I cried when I didn't listen. I wanted to cry to Rafe, but I really couldn't call him twenty-seven times in one day. He had stuff to do. His sister was, apparently, a handful. His mother also. He even admitted to losing patience with me. I still called him a dozen times a day. Once, when he was out, I kept trying late into the night until his mother finally took the phone off the hook. I got scared that the receiver would never be replaced, I'd never get through to Rafe again, and I was up all night frightened and shaking and listening to the busy signal over and over again. But mostly when I'd call, he was there but in the middle of something or cross or preoccupied, and when I asked if he still loved me, he'd scream, *Yes! Now, will you just leave me alone!* He hated me for being so fucked up right when he needed to deal with a life that had more in it than me.

I realized I'd better do something, get a hold of myself because no one else would. I announced to my mother that I thought I should go to Dallas for a friend's wedding. I told her I needed her to pay for my ticket, but I'd give the money back because when I got down there I'd write some articles for the *Morning News* and make the trip profitable. She thought that the need to run from place to place was a bad one, a sign of my sickness, and agreed only on the condition that Dr. Sterling said it was okay. Dr. Sterling was away for Christmas, but that hadn't kept me from calling her at 4:00 in the morning several times at her ski lodge up in Vermont, so I didn't see why my mom couldn't call her at the same place during the day. Thank God, Dr. Sterling felt that traveling or doing whatever would keep me going until I got back to Cambridge and back into treatment was a fine idea because she'd been talking to me for the last few days and she'd never heard me sound quite this desperate.

What neither of them knew was that I was planning a layover in Minneapolis on my way back from Dallas so I could see Rafe and make sure he still loved me.

So I went to Texas, I made some pretense of writing articles. I showed up at the *Morning News* and took my old desk because everyone was on vacation and the few remaining editors were starved for copy. I interviewed people, I planned to write something about a couple of Texas writers whose books had just been published, but once I finished making transcripts, I realized I didn't have it in me to write.

Every time I talked to my mother, I told her it was all fine and good down here, that I was writing a lot, being paid by the piece, earning my keep, that this was the best thing I'd ever done.

I spent the rest of the time in Dallas in bed, emerging only on New Year's Eve to see *Broadcast News*, and it seemed ridiculous that the Holly Hunter character reserved fifteen minutes every morning to cry when I couldn't reserve a time not to cry all day.

Rafe was late to meet me at the airport. When he finally showed up, he found me sobbing in the Continental terminal and started explaining about how his alarm clock was broken.

I wanted to kill him because I took a 6:00 A.M. flight and changed planes in Houston so I could see him, and now he's talking to me about how household appliances made in Japan are defective and I can't believe he wasn't up all night waiting for me the way I would have been for him. But I didn't say that, realizing in some tiny little sane corner of my brain that I am crazy and he probably isn't.

I sat there and cried all the way into Minneapolis, and Rafe said we'd talk when I was calm.

In a restaurant, he told me he couldn't stay in the relationship, I need him too much, and so do all these other people, and he just wanted to be a normal senior in college who enjoys his last term before graduation and drops a lot of acid and fucks a lot of random freshman women and doesn't have to worry about someone like me.

I didn't respond because I thought I might be dead.

I was supposed to be in Minneapolis only for the afternoon, I was supposed to get on a flight to New York in a few hours, but I refused to board an airplane until Rafe changed his mind.

So we went to his house, I met his mother with her thick German accent and her severe Prussian manner, and we drank white wine and took pictures as if everything were fine, and I conveniently missed my flight. I was so quiet and well behaved that Rafe decided we didn't have to break up after all. Later on, after we'd taken Rafe's sister to see *The Empire of the Sun*, the kid flipped out and gouged a hole in the foyer wall with a *New York Times* umbrella, the kind you get free with home delivery. They took her to the emergency room in the middle of the night because she wouldn't calm down, she wouldn't stop doing violence to the infrastructure of her mother's grand old home overlooking Lake Minnetonka, and it looked like they were going to have to commit her.

I was left alone in the house, alone in the guest room in the Minneapolis dark, and I was so frightened that I called Dr. Sterling.

"I'll be on a flight to New York tomorrow," I tell her after I've explained where I am. "Rafe and I have patched things up, but I don't know. I've a feeling it might not last."

"You sound okay about that," she says.

"I am right now, because I'm still here." I pause for a minute to try to figure out why I don't sound more upset. "Let's face it, it's five in the morning and I'm calling you, so I can't be that okay."

"I think you should come back up to Cambridge right away, and we need to think about some very aggressive form of treatment. I'm worried about what's happened to you over the last few weeks. And you're always saying, 'What do I have to do to get people to take me seriously?' Well, listen, you don't have to try to kill yourself first. I take you seriously now. I think I might be able to arrange with Stillman or one of the other Harvard hospitals to have you checked in as a full-time patient, with me supervising your case through one of the doctors I know there."

I'm silent. I'm stunned.

"But the first thing you've got to do is get back here where I can see you. I can't be much help by phone."

"Dr. Sterling?" I whimper.

"Yes?"

"Thanks."

10

Blank Girl

* * *

I myself am hell
ROBERT LOWELL
"Skunk Hour"

It is a Saturday night in January and I am lying in a bed in the infirmary, watching television. I am also reading Margaret Atwood's book *Surfacing*, even though it is hopelessly polemic and dated, hoping it will awaken my feminist consciousness, hoping it will inspire me to want to get out of bed and go out to the wilderness and explore my relationship with the earth and tree roots and sheep and my own naked, unshowered, unadorned self, which is what the narrator in the story does. By the end of the book, she is covered in mud, a real live natural woman, burying her own shit in dirt, as if *that* is what it's all about. I am going to have to inform my friends, all of them right-minded women who think they should read *Surfacing* because it's supposed to be a feminist classic, not to bother.

Maybe what I really need is some Thoreau, *Walden* perhaps, since everyone says that it will make me happy to be alive. Henry David puttering around in his garden and all that.

Not that I can even aspire to happiness anymore. I am just hoping that something can show me that there is a way to live that is so satisfying and fulfilling in and of itself that I won't even want Rafe anymore. I would like, so much, to be one of those independent women like Barbara Stanwyck in *Baby Face* or Jean Harlow in *Red-Headed Woman* or any *film noir* star in any old movie who can love 'em and leave 'em with impunity. Unfortunately, in the blue-and-white-striped cotton pajamas that are the Stillman uniform, I am just me.

The U.S. Figure Skating Championship is on TV, so I watch the various competitors do their routines, listening to the sportscasters make references to back camels and triple jumps and high leaps. It is the women who are competing tonight. The only ones I've heard of are Tiffany Chin, the delicate Asian girl who is doomed to take second place to Debi Thomas, the Stanford premed who is doomed to give a lousy performance at the Olympics and walk away with just a bronze medal.

Debi is kind of chunky, not in any way pretty, nothing at all like the figure skaters I always idolized and fell in love with when I was little. They were always lithe, lean, if not beautiful like Peggy Fleming then adorable and charming in a pixyish way like Dorothy Hamill. I know that skating is supposed to be about pirouettes on ice, about double toe loops and triple axels and not feminine beauty, but I am as seduced as anyone by the superficial side of it, and can still remember going to the Ice Capades at Madison Square Garden year after year, dreaming on and on about growing up to be Peggy Fleming. She especially was blessed with blue eyes and black hair and a dancer's lankiness that was never again duplicated by an American skater, never again repeated at all until Katarina Witt.

It is not until later, much later, through confessional articles in *People* magazine, that I learn that all these women suffer the loneliness of the road, the stress of having to stay in shape, the difficulty of being a professional athlete. It is at the same time that I discover that many of the pretty ballerinas in *Swan Lake*, the beautiful but not quite unique models who wait on tables and do occasional spreads in *Glamour*, the tennis champions, the girl backup singers—that all these women who seem to be in enviable positions are in fact mired in misery.

Even Debi Thomas has her own problems. She will eventually transfer to the less competitive University of Colorado, get married, and give up skating altogether. But on this particular night, she delivers a transcendent performance, completing all those triple flips, twisting through all those back camels, making all those grand leaps, getting the sportscasters to gush about how she's in top form, how she's really been gearing up for this meet for a while—and would you look at her do all those jumps in tandem! Debi, for tonight, is a star. She has no grace, but she is strong and solid, traits that seem especially admirable as I lie in bed, weak and unstable.

I too get carried away with the joy of Debi's moment. She smiles as she skates, looking so confident, and I think, To hell with *Surfacing* and the Cro-Magnon woman's existence, it is figure skating, the mastery of metal blades on thin ice, that is what living is about. I know from my own dance lessons that it is taxing and exhausting to get to the point where your dancing is actually enjoyable, to arrive at a place where the mind no longer has to concentrate on when to *relevé*, when to do the *pas de deux*. It takes years of practice for the limbs to develop an internal memory. But when they do, when the body takes over, it feels like freedom, like *dancing* instead of just dancing. So I watch Debi skate, knowing all the hard work and the years of training that lead up to this one performance (and to others, but this is the only one that counts right now), and I start to cry.

I think I am crying tears of joy because there is beauty in seeing this young woman, my age approximately, giving this exhilarating performance. I cry when I look at her smile. Because she smiles as she skates, knowing that she is doing everything right and that this is the right thing for her to do. And I am still crying when she ascends the center platform in the winners' circle, the high one above the two lower pedestals for the bronze and silver medalists, to receive her gold pendant. I cry, and Debi cries too. This triumph proves that her bad luck at the Olympics hasn't ruined her and that, as the sportscasters mention with undue gravity, her loss to Tiffany Chin at the U.S. Championships last year was just a fluke.

I am still crying long after the broadcast is over, and I realize these are not tears of joy at all. These are, in fact, the same tears I cry when I see Gorbachev on the nightly news and know that this man has changed the world as we know it and that he proves that one man can make a difference. These are the same tears I cry when I hear the gospel song that goes *This little light of mine, I'm gonna make it shine*, and I think of the way that ordinary people are able to triumph, in ways small and large, over adversity.

And I remember being in junior high and crying this way for hours after seeing Robert Redford in *The Natural*, crying over the way determination and conviction can make a simple baseball player do supernatural things. The tears pour down after the movie as I eat dinner with my mother at Sbarro in Times Square on Friday evening, and she demands to know what I am so upset about. And all I can say, over and over again, is that he's a natural, he's a natural, it's such a gift to be a natural, it is such a responsibility, it is so hard to be a natural.

And then my mother says, because she seems to understand, "You relate to this, Ellie, don't you?"

I nod my head yes.

"You relate to this because you're a natural too?"

Yes, I want to tell her, and maybe I even do say that, but I am crying because whatever my gifts, the pieces of good buried inside and under so much that I feel is bad, is wrong, is twisted, are less clear than the ability to hit a ball with a bat and break the scoreboard or do a triple pirouette in the air on ice. My gifts are for life itself, for an unfortunately astute understanding of all the cruelty and pain in the world. My gifts are unspecific. I am an artist manqué, someone full of crazy ideas and grandiloquent needs and even a little bit of happiness, but with no particular way to express it. I am like the title character in the film *Betty Blue*, the woman who is so full of . . . so full of . . . so full of something or other—it is unclear what, but a definite energy that can't find its medium—who pokes her own eyes out with a scissors and is murdered by her lover in an insane asylum in the end. She is, and I am becoming, a complete waste. So I cry at the end of *The Natural*.

And here I am, years later, when it is supposed to be clear that I am a writer, that it is through words that I will escape this sense of having no art form, and it is Saturday night, and instead of being out at a party in Adams House or seeing a double feature of Preston Sturges flicks at the Brattle Theatre or just smoking grass with my friends, I am lying in bed in the infirmary watching TV.

This is, I remind myself, all I can do right now. I am depressed to the point of being incapable of much else besides lying in this white room with these white sheets and white blankets, watching a television set suspended from the ceiling which changes channels with a remote control that you squeeze like a lemon that might be souring your tea. I know I can do so much more than this, I know that I could be a life force, could love with a heart full of soul, could feel with the power that flies men to the moon. I know that if I could just get out from under this depression, there is so much I could do besides cry in front of the TV on a Saturday night.

Dr. Sterling agrees, when I first check into the infirmary, that I can lie there for as long as I like, but I need to get my work done. Always, always, no matter how bad life seems to be, I must hand in my papers on time or take my finals when I am supposed to or meet deadlines for stories. So my word processor and all my books make the trek to Stillman with me, where I entertain fantasies of finding solace in my studies as I was once able to do.

But I'm too far gone for that now. It seems that I have spent so much time trying to convince people that I really am depressed, that I really can't cope—but now that it's finally true, I don't want to admit it. I am petrified by what is happening to me, so frightened of what the bottom of the well will look like once I sink down there, so frightened that in fact this is it. How did this happen to me? It seems not so long ago, maybe only a decade ago, I was a little girl trying out a new persona, trying on morbid depression as some kind of punk rock statement, and now here I am, the real thing.

I find myself calling Dr. Sterling every five minutes to get her to assure and reassure me that I will come out of this one day. And she always does, always says the right things. But a few seconds after I hang up, I'm frightened all over again. So I call all over again.

"Elizabeth, we just went through this," she says. "What can I do to make you believe me?"

"You can't," I say through tears. "Don't you get it? Nothing sticks. That's my whole problem. Rafe leaves the room for five minutes, and I'm sure he's never coming back.

And that's how it is for me with everything. Nothing is real to me unless it's right in front of me."

"What a terrible way to live."

"That's what I'm trying to tell you!"

I wonder if she understands that I can't go on like this.

And still, I keep telling myself that recovery is an act of will, that if I decide one day that I simply must get up and out of this bed, that I must be happy, I will be able to force it to happen. Why do I believe this is possible?

I suppose because the alternative is too frightening. The alternative will lead to my inevitable suicide. Up until now, I always thought of self-destructive behavior as a red flag to wave at the world, a way of getting the help I needed. But the truth is, lying here in Stillman, for the first time ever I am contemplating suicide completely seriously, because this pain is too much. I wonder if all the nurses who traipse through here to bring me meals, to change the sheets, to remind me to shower—I wonder if any of them can tell from just looking at me that all I am is the sum total of my pain, a raw wound-edness so extreme that it might be terminal. It might be terminal velocity, the speed of the sound of a girl falling down to a place from where she can't be retrieved. What if I am stuck down here for good?

I call Dr. Sterling again, ask her the same questions again, and she decides, finally, that I must be given some kind of drug. After all, I am not her only patient, I am not her only problem, and every time she says something to me about feeling like she really needs to spend time with her children, I start to cry and tell her that if I die, there will be blood on her hands. If for no reason other than that she wants her private life back, Dr. Sterling is willing to try a chemical cure. She thinks that with the right medication, I might even be able to get my work done. Both my academic adviser and Dr. Sterling, along with several friends, have suggested that I just take incompletes in my courses and make up the work some other time, but for some reason, I just can't. It would be too demoralizing. If I can write my papers, I keep telling myself, then I'll know that I don't yet have to abandon all hope. I know that if I don't do my schoolwork, I really will be compelled to kill myself because the last bit of what I have to hold on to will be gone. Other kids with emotional troubles take time off from school, but they have families, they have some sense of a place in this world that can absorb them in all their pain; all I have is the semblance of a life that I have made for myself here at Harvard, and I can't let go of it. I *must* do my work.

My main symptoms, Dr. Sterling believes, are anxiety and agitation. In her opinion, even worse than the depression itself is the fear I seem to have about never escaping from it. As usual, my problem seems to be that I am one step removed from my problems, more a nervous audience member at a horror movie than the movie itself. "So you think I'm suffering from meta-depression?" I ask Dr. Sterling in a moment of humor.

"That's one way to see it," she replies.

Dr. Sterling believes that the best drug for me, at least until I go for a thorough evaluation with a psychopharmacologist at McLean, is Xanax, mainly because it will have an immediate effect. An antidepressant might ultimately be a more appropriate antidote for my ills, but Dr. Sterling doesn't think I'll live to see the results of that kind of drug, which will take a few weeks to kick in, if we don't find a solution to my immediate desperation.

Some time after taking my first Xanax, after going for my daily constitutional, I am back in my bed at Stillman, curled up tight, my arms squeezing my pillow, convinced that I am permanently stuck in this miserable morass. Life is awful, life has always been awful, life will always be awful. In fact, with every passing day it is getting worse and worse. Dr. Sterling calls to check up on me. I tell her that while I was out in the square, standing on an interminably long line at Au Bon Pain, I nearly had a panic attack, nearly collapsed and had a convulsion in the middle of a fast-food café because I felt so suffocated. I start yelling about how she'd told me that Xanax was good for anxiety disorders, but I had never felt so nervous in my life. I tell her that I am clinging to my pillow because I am certain that the men in white coats are going to come in here and take me away any minute now, and if I hold on tightly enough maybe they won't put me in a straitjacket.

"Elizabeth," she says, laughing, "you're already exactly where those men in white would take you, so there's no danger of that happening. Sounds like you had a negative reaction to the Xanax." She's so matter-of-fact, as if I were not in the midst of a psychosomatic emergency.

"I think that maybe it relaxed me so much that I was actually relaxed enough to think about my problems in an uninhibited fashion," I suggest. "Which made me realize how much I was kidding myself, which made me realize that my life is even worse than even I thought."

"Listen," Dr. Sterling responds, "I really don't think you should be taking the Xanax anymore. I think we're going to have to find something else."

As soon as we hang up, against the doctor's orders, I take a few more hits of Xanax, hoping that they'll put me to sleep long enough for the bad feelings to go away. But it doesn't quite work out that way. True, I do manage to go to sleep for a good long time. But all night I dream of walls closing in on me, of being a wild animal caught in a trap by fur hunters, so desperate to get away that I bite off my own leg and instead of escaping, I bleed to death in the snow. The ground is red, the ground is white, the sky is blue, and when I wake up the bad feelings do not go away.

Often, in movies and novels, a favorite character is the devoted therapist, the one who goes swimming with his crazy patient to prove to her that she isn't going to drown just because her older sister did, or the one who flies across the country and meets the whole family to figure out why her pathetic charge is such a twisted young man. Of course, another stock character is the evil, manipulative psychiatrist, the Hannibal Lecter who kills his irritating, untreatable manic-depressive patient and then eats the flesh of his carcass with fava beans and Chianti. Most of my therapists have been closer to the latter type, although their cannibalism was strictly metaphorical. Dr. Sterling is the only psychiatrist about whom I can truly say, She saved my life. I think she knew that she probably wasn't going to be paid for all of her efforts, but she did what she felt was necessary anyway.

In fact, with my explicit permission, she even got in touch with my father, though I told her that under no circumstances would I talk to him myself. I think she was partly curious to speak with him, as she had heard so much about him over the last few months. But mostly she seemed to believe that if his insurance really did cover ninety percent of the cost of therapy, there had to be some way to get him to pitch in. During that stay at Stillman, she called my father and told him that she understood that he had all sorts of reasons why he felt it was up to my mother to pay for my therapy, and perhaps, she said—humoring him, no doubt—in less dire straits that might have been a reasonable decision on his part, but she really needed to see me every day, and she wanted to know that he would pay for what my mother couldn't. I don't know exactly what else ensued, but she must have made the situation sound extremely desperate, because it worked. Within a week, he mailed off some insurance forms for Dr. Sterling to fill out.

Dr. Sterling succeeded in inventing a type of asylum for me within the Harvard medical system, sparing me a stint at a full-service mental institution. Because I'd briefly been some version of okay when we first commenced treatment, Dr. Sterling knew that somewhere in my personality there was a giggly girl who just wanted to have fun, and she thought it was important that I be allowed to express that aspect of myself. She seemed to think that one fine day I might come into my exuberant self again, and that at McLean I'd have only mattressed wallpaper and iron-barred windows and the schizophrenic down the hall to indulge it with. Her goal was to see to it that I got the kind of care and treatment that I would have at a psychiatric hospital without actually being placed in such complete confinement. It is only because of her determination and dedication that I survived that year without actually being committed, and it is only because of her that I am alive today at all.

I tried to remind myself that Rafe was not the problem. The problem, as Dr. Sterling explained it to me and as I myself knew, was that I was fucked up. Rafe was merely a makeshift solution I'd come up with, a pill I took to make the bad feelings go away. But now that he was not cooperating so well, now that he was refusing to be used this way, now that he was insisting that he wanted to be my boyfriend and not my panacea, he was no longer part of the solution. He was part of the problem.

Story of my life: I am so self-destructive, I turn solutions into problems. Everything I touch, I ruin. I'm Midas in reverse.

Before I could even begin to contemplate the big issues of my day—to shampoo or not to shampoo, that is the question—Alden walked in, armed with some clothing that I'd asked for, and a cup of hot chocolate from Au Bon Pain, which I thanked her for. I didn't want to ask if anyone had called because I didn't want to be disappointed, and I'm sure that if Rafe rang, she'd have told me. It was, after all, Alden who always left those big Magic Marker notes saying, "Rafe called," or sometimes just "He called." Although her message-taking skills were otherwise lackadaisical, Alden knew when a call was important.

So I didn't ask and she didn't mention anything and the day went on and people came by. Susannah brought me a copy of Joni Mitchell's *The Hissing of Summer Lawns* because I wanted to see the words to "Don't Interrupt the Sorrow," and she told me that I should really be reading P. G. Wodehouse or J. P. Donleavy, something cheerful and humorous. Paul came by and brought me Chinese food and a vanilla-scented candle, and we went for a walk in the snow to his apartment on Mt. Auburn Street and listened to *Clouds* on his portable tape player. Jonathan, the managing editor of the *Crimson*, came by with an anthology of female erotic fiction, the *Village Voice*, and the latest *New Republic*. Samantha came by with a copy of Paul Johnson's *Modern Times*, which she said somehow related to how I was feeling. I kept hoping someone would bring me the latest *Cosmopolitan* so I could read my horoscope and find out if my life was ever going to work out again, but no one did.

And the day went on until the evening came, and my long-term fantasy about lying in a hospital bed and receiving visitors had turned into a reality, and it was all very nice and good, but nothing mattered if Rafe didn't call. Eben and Alec came by with a chocolate milk shake from Steve's and a turkey and boursin sandwich from Formaggio, and I had a nice time talking to them, but already when they arrived I was starting to get hazy. And however well rested and well liked I was feeling, it was no deterrent to the sense of crazy that started traveling all through my body, and up into my head until I felt suffocated with it as if I were buried naked and alive in hot white summer sand, burning to death.

And finally, there is no one left to visit me, no Alden,

no Paul, no Susannah, no Samantha, no Jonathan, no Eben, no Alec, nobody, and there is no one left to buffer the pain, the tremendous pain, the great big fucking pain, and I start to cry. And all I can think is, *Why hasn't Rafe called he's disappearing he's leaving me like everyone else he promised he wouldn't but he is I know it oh my God I want to die right here right now in this adjustable infirmary bed I want my corpse to be white like these sheets whiter than these blankets I want to be drained of my blood and my humanity forever I never want to feel again.*

And the crying and the pain that goes with it becomes too much to bear. Usually, tears are cathartic. As you cry, the salt and water shed from your eyes and drag misery along the way. But in this case, the crying only escalates the emotions that it expresses, and the more I cry, the more upset I get, and I am thinking of every time I cried over Rafe, every time I cried because I thought he didn't love me well enough, and every time he would reassure me and tell me I was being silly, but now I am realizing that I was not being silly, because where is he now, where is he as I lay dying, and why is it that no one who is supposed to be here for me ever is?

And pretty soon the crying is about Daddy leaving, about being alone in my crib, being alone in my mother's womb, being alone in this life, and I know that I have been hysterical many times before, but this time, I don't think it's going to stop. Somebody has to make this stop! I wonder if the Xanax will help, wonder if I still have some hidden in my knapsack, wonder if anything will work or if there is no pill, no potion, no serum, no shot, nothing under the whole big black sun that can possibly penetrate a pain so deep. Well, there must be something, some very strong hand with a very tight grip that can turn off the crazy way I feel.

So I call Dr. Sterling. I start screaming at her about my lack of clarity and my fear. And then I tell her that I think I will try to call Rafe sometime tomorrow morning, and I wish there was something that would knock me out until then. In fact, I continue, I wish something would knock me out for a long time until the way I feel just stops, because this is not even an issue for therapy anymore. We can analyze it for days and that won't take away the pain. Something bigger than me is taking over my body and mind. I'm possessed.

Dr. Sterling asks me to be more specific about what's wrong and what it would take to make me feel better. I keep repeating that I want my brain annihilated, that it won't stop running and churning and burning and trying to make sense of my life, and even here in the infirmary, it still needs a vacation. I think I finally say, I want my head blotted out. I want heroin. Of course, Dr. Sterling won't prescribe a narcotic for me. Instead she decides to put me on a drug called Mellaril, an antipsychotic, a medication that's been known to help schizophrenics during their visionary episodes, a major tranquilizer in the same family as Thorazine. It is, she assures me, a complete brain drain, and it will most certainly knock me out.

After I hang up the phone, still crying like a rainstorm, a nurse walks in and gives me a small brown tablet and some cranberry juice, sort of the house drink at Stillman. She tells me to be careful not to choke since she sees that I'm wheezing from so much crying.

And quite amazingly, only a few minutes after I swallow the Mellaril, my tears and all my feelings completely subside. Just like that. Like magic. I am calm, carefree, careless. I sit there in my bed staring at the wall, feeling happy, enjoying the way the wall looks, how pink and how white it is. Pink and white, as far as I'm concerned, have never looked quite so pink and white before.

The next day, Dr. Sterling announces that she is so pleased with the effect Mellaril has had on me, she's decided it ought to be my drug of choice. Three times a day, the nurse will give me a little brown tablet.

I'm not sure what she wants the medication's effect to be. Apparently some doctors at McLean are experimenting with low dosages as an antidepressant. But its main result is my complete indifference to everything. After the initial euphoria I experienced with my first dose, a standard regimen of Mellaril just dulls everything. Instead of being Depressed Girl, I'm Blank Girl. I achieve a lack of affect so complete that Dr. Sterling and the other physicians almost mistake it for an improvement. And I guess it is: I am calm enough to write a semiotics paper, calm enough to compose an essay for my tutorial about feminist theory and *The Oresteia Trilogy*, calm enough to contemplate going home for a few days during intercession.

I call Rafe, who announces that the plans we'd made to meet for a few days in New York before he goes back to Brown won't work because he needs to write some papers and do other things so he can graduate. I hear him, but his words don't register. It's as if the Mellaril has blocked the receptor sites in my brain which connect facts with feelings.

Someone could walk into this room and say your life is on fire, I hear Paul Simon singing in some song somewhere in a life that seems so far away.

11

Good Morning Heartache

✳ ✳ ✳

I'm going out of my mind
With a pain that stops and starts
Like a corkscrew through my heart
Ever since we've been apart
BOB DYLAN
"You're a Big Girl Now"

I showed up on Rafe's doorstep unannounced when I knew
he'd been back at Brown for a week and I still hadn't heard
from him. After he broke up with me, he didn't even have
the decency to escort me to the bus station because he had
play rehearsal and couldn't get away. Instead he had his roommate drive me there. I felt like a sickly visiting relative that
everyone grudgingly takes turns attending to because it would
be wrong not to. I had images of Rafe saying to this roommate, I don't want to deal with her; you do it.

We got into his little Honda, it was below freezing, and
I kept thinking I ought to be grateful, if Rafe had taken me
to the bus, we'd have had to walk, but somehow I didn't feel
that way. The roommate deposited me at the bus depot, all
awkwardness, because what do you say to someone you're
never going to see again for reasons that have nothing to do
with anything that's transpired between the two of you? And
it took all the strength I could muster to purchase a ticket,

get on board, get a seat, buy some magazines for the road even though I couldn't concentrate on anything at all. Couldn't concentrate on the *Premiere* cover story about Cher. Or the *New York* article on John Cassablancas and his modeling agency. Couldn't even get through the contents page in *Cosmopolitan*. Couldn't even concentrate on Rafe, because how can you focus on something so consuming that it's everywhere, like the air? The only thing I could do was go blank. And I remember thinking: *This is it. This is the pain you've been waiting for all your life. Heartbreak straight up.* I remember thinking things couldn't be worse.

Everyone has relationships in college that go on for a few months and then just fall apart, in the way that these things do. Sometimes the end hurts bad, sometimes it's no big deal, sometimes it's a pleasant relief, but mostly it's nothing that a few days of sitting on a friend's couch with a box of tissues and a bottle of gin can't cure.

Anyone looking on from the outside would have deposited my involvement with Rafe into that slush pile of short-term loves that don't quite take off. Anyone who didn't know the particulars would have said we were a young couple with youth, timing, and distance as the preeminent factors preventing the relationship from enduring beyond the first ninety days. We were incompatible, geographically challenged, not ready for commitment—those would be among the usual litany of excuses for our demise, and they would even be the stock answers I would give to people who asked, innocently enough, Whatever happened to that Rafe guy? And no one would have any reason to doubt me. Anyone who didn't know better could never have imagined what an intense folie à deux we had come to inhabit during our brief union.

Rafe took it upon himself to absorb my anguish completely. Part of what he liked about me was that I was depressed. He was like one of those people who is terminally attracted to alcoholics or drug addicts, only in my case I was an abuser without a substance.

At times he relished the idea of being my personal Jesus, of setting up a safe haven for me in his little house in Providence, Rhode Island. I would lie in his bed for days on end, and he would bring me toast and tea and tell me he loved me and ask me to talk to him about my pain. He liked the idea of salvation. His mother was a high-maintenance hysteric, his younger sister was some version of a pre-adolescent psychotic, and Rafe's natural role in life was as caretaker.

It's not that unusual. Throughout the ages, troubled individuals with a knack for self-preservation have mated themselves to people who groove on their pain, knowing it's the best chance they've got to find love and care. I mean, who else but a voyeur of misery would have put up with me during my deepest depression? I got lucky when Rafe found me. And in my short dating career, I've taken up with three different guys who, at the time I met them, had girlfriends in mental hospitals. Surely that can't be normal, can't be a claim every girl can make. At the point of initial attraction, I didn't know that these men tended to fall for crazy women and they didn't know that I was the very thing, and still we sniffed each other out, sensed the odor of a certain cerebral mutation, saw each other across crowded rooms and made introductions because some things are just meant to be: Sid will always find Nancy; Tom will always hook up with Roseanne; and Ted (truly a reprobate case) will manage to get involved, in tandem, with both Sylvia and another woman who died with her head in the oven. F. Scott will always recognize his Zelda; Samson will always fall for Delilah; and Jason would wed Medea all over again, even if he were fully apprised of their marriage's macabre denouement. Do I detect a pattern here?

But until Rafe, I'd never been one of the lucky ones. I was always single, with occasional lapses into—well, into other kinds of lapses. I would hear about other girls who'd gone mad and been locked away, and I'd hear how they had these mournful, devoted boyfriends who would wipe their noses, tie old rags and bandannas around their bloodied wrists, run out to the pharmacy to get a last-minute prescription for a sedative called in by the doctor as the girl had a psychotic episode right there on the kitchen floor. I'd hear about these girls and wonder how they could have suffered so when they were so loved. Isolation and a sense that all human connection was elusive, was the province of others, of the happy people on the other side of the glass wall, was the worst part of my depression. I used to think: I want in on whatever deal it is that these other fucked-up chicks have got!

And then Rafe came along, and he tried to love me, I really believe he did, but there was no amount of love that would have stitched my wounded psyche at that point. In fact, compared to all the other forces at work in the world, love is rather impotent and pitiful: My father must have told me a million times how much he loved me, but that emotion—assuming it was even real—hardly had the strength to counter the many other acts of wrong he committed against me. Contrary to romance novels and the love-conquers-all mentality that even those of us who grew up in an era of divorce are—in response to some atavistic instinct—still raised to believe, love is always a product and a victim of circumstances. It is fragile and small. As Leonard Cohen once wrote, "Love is not a victory march / It's a cold and it's a broken hallelujah." I discovered, through the love Rafe gave me, that affection as medicine is highly overrated, that a person who is as sick with depression as I most certainly was cannot possibly be rescued through the power of anyone's love. It is just so much worse than that. I mean, if you were to find a shattered mirror, find all the pieces, all the shards and all the tiny chips, and have whatever skill and patience it took to put all that broken glass back together so that it was complete once again, the restored mirror would still be spiderwebbed with cracks, it would still be a useless glued version of its former self, which could show only fragmented reflections of anyone looking into it. Some things are beyond repair. And that was me: There was so much damage, it was going to take a lot more than one person, or even one therapist, one drug, one electric shock treatment—it was going to take a lot of everything before the Humpty Dumpty remains of my life could be reassembled. It would have taken—and eventually did take—so much more than Rafe to save me.

And instead, his indulgence actually made me worse. A psychologist once explained to me that the worst thing a therapist can do to an extremely depressed patient is be nice. Because that kindness creates a stasis, allows the depressive to remain comfortable in her current miserable state. In order for therapy to be effective, a patient must be prodded and provoked, forced into confrontations, given sufficient incentive to push herself out of the caged fog of depression. Rafe was probably too nice to me. He allowed me to feel bad and that, in turn, allowed me to feel even worse. All I ever did with Rafe was wallow in my pain.

In striking contrast, Nathan, my boyfriend after Rafe and after I was a whole lot better, did not suffer my depressive episodes gladly. In fact, he hated them—they were the thing about me that he liked the least, and by the time we started dating, in 1988, there actually was a lot more to me. I was still given to running out of doors and crying on the front lawn. I was still (and probably always will be) a person who made scenes when I got upset. But Nathan handled these situations much differently from Rafe. He would say, Come on, this is ridiculous. He would say, Enough already. He would say, Snap out of it. And you know what? His approach worked. Forced to behave, I behaved; forced to cope, I coped. By that time, of course, I had the tools with which to manage my emotions more efficiently, but still, I think Nathan's way was better than Rafe's. In the years I was with Nathan, I thrived, while with Rafe I just deteriorated. This is not to say that either of these men were Svengali enough to have controlled me. And I'm sure I chose each of them for their respective qualities and how they jibed with the state I was in at those two very different times of my life. But still I have no doubt that Rafe's eagerness to be there for me while I was hurting encouraged me to hurt more. Of course it did: I wanted so badly to please him.

At a certain point, he realized he couldn't cope with it. I un-

*derstand his decision, I really do. I understood it even at the time.
But it didn't make it hurt any less.*

How can you do this to me? *I kept asking when we sat on
his bedroom floor and talked, as we sat there for hours one Saturday
afternoon breaking up.* You let me be myself, you encouraged
me to let you see how terrible I felt inside, you let me get
more and more sad and hysterical, and now that I'm as low
as I'm ever going to be, you're leaving me.

*That's right, he said. He couldn't lie. He told me he thought
he could handle it, but he couldn't. He thought a lot of things. He
never meant to hurt me.*

*I didn't, at the time, say to him that he loved watching me get
hysterical, got off on it, enjoyed the* mise en scène, *the emotional
rawness. I didn't say it because I didn't have to. It was obvious. He
was always telling me that my purity, my complete inability to mask
my sense of horror, was what he loved about me most. It was like he
didn't understand that those qualities, at least in me, were a pathology. My rawness was not in any way about purity—it was about
depression. Yes, there was a certain beautiful honesty to my depressed
state—I miss it sometimes now. I miss having so little stake in
maintaining the status quo that I could walk out of rooms in tears at
times that other people would have deemed inappropriate. I liked that
about myself. I liked that disregard for convention. And Rafe, well,
Rafe loved it.*

*But it was sick, sicker than even he knew at first. The purity
turned into perversity. It turned not into just an awareness of the
darkness, but a morbid obsession with it. And as soon as he figured
that out, he bolted. He left me alone with my depression, having
exhausted him and every other last resort I had.*

Before I left Providence, I called my friend Archer to tell him
that I was coming into New York, that I was feeling crazy
and desperate, that I would come straight to his apartment,
that he had to provide me with a decent dinner because I

couldn't take care of myself. And he said in his Waspy, courteous way something like, Sure, come on over.

Archer is what you call a real straight arrow, a Boston Brahmin to the manner born. He pretty much wanted everything to be simple and pleasant. The blood and squalor of life that keeps the majority of us intrigued and tantalized held no appeal for Archer. After we saw *Casualties of War* together, a movie where Sean Penn and Michael J. Fox play soldiers whose squadron in Vietnam rapes and beats a poor peasant girl to death, Archer just kept asking me what the point was to sitting through all that messy sordidness. Let's just say that Broadway musicals like *Annie* and *Oklahoma!* were probably invented with people like Archer in mind. He was positively dapper. After Archer graduated from Harvard in 1987, he got a job working for American Express doing God-knows-what (something about the database for the travel division, he once told me), and it is only because he is picture-perfect handsome that Archer has amassed a stable of vibrant, nutty women into his coterie. He's one of those Yankee gentlemen who collects hysterical Jewesses as good buddies because we are as foreign and exotic to him as the natives in Tahiti were to Gauguin— and no matter how well he got to know any of us, his bafflement never abated. Everything kind of slides by Archer: I honestly believe that when the rain falls down, it never lands on him. If Archer weren't so good-looking, I'm not sure he'd exist at all, since he lacks most vital signs. But his pulchritude is almost part of the problem: Archer is so flawlessly handsome that he actually seems sterile, possessed of such a pure and symmetrical beauty that it is devoid of the Eros and Thanatos and virility that would make a man less physically endowed far more appealing. Basically, Archer is the perfect guy to go see after a breakup because he is the best opportunity to hang out with a gorgeous man and be certain that there will be no sexual tension whatsoever.

That night, Archer takes me to a lovely dinner at a lovely restaurant called Brandywine and remains perfectly unaware the whole time that I'm communicating with him from behind a blurry, opaque glass, kind of like a bathroom window. He is conversing with me about his plans to move to Zurich, why he's a registered Republican, where he gets his shirts dry-cleaned, and all the while I am full of this terrible pain so deep that I dare not let it near the surface. As I step back from my own self-absorption, it seems suddenly incredible to me that I am quaking inside, that, emotionally speaking, I am an avalanche that's about to land, in rocks and pebbles and stones, at Archer's feet, and he is still managing to engage me in a discussion of the presidential primaries. Every so often, I space out and say, I'm sorry, I got distracted, what did you just say? And a couple of times I come very close to saying, Can't you see I'm a mess?! Why don't you ask me why?

But I stay silent. The whole point of Archer is that he doesn't ask, he is a mannequin with a few human functions. That night I sleep in the same bed as Archer. He pulls me close at first, but I migrate to the opposite end and cling to the corner like somebody hanging over the side of a tall building, about to slip off the edge.

Sometimes, I get so consumed by depression that it is hard to believe that the whole world doesn't stop and suffer with me.

I couldn't move after Rafe left me. Really. I was stuck to my bed like a piece of chewing gum at the bottom of somebody's shoe, branded to the underside, adhering to someone who didn't want me, who kept stamping on me but still I wouldn't move away. I couldn't get unstuck. I lay there, gobbling down my Mellaril at regular intervals, wondering why even the dulling effects of this stupefying drug were not strong enough to help me.

At first, I was staying at my mother's house in New York, but eventually I went back to Cambridge because Dr. Sterling thought it would be better if I were close to the center of treatment (i.e., her). It was pretty much the same to me either way. The one big difference was that in New York there was an abundance of food in the kitchen and in Cambridge there was nothing; hence, at home I ate sparingly and listlessly, but at school I just plain starved. Either way, I seemed to be fading.

While I was still in my old room at home, I discovered that the hardest part of each day, as is the case with most depressives, was simply getting out of bed in the morning. If I could do that much I had a fighting chance. To get through the day, that is. I decided to try to do some writing, hoping it might afford me the same sense of release that it once had, so many years before. But as soon as I sat down at my typewriter, I froze before the keyboard. I couldn't think of a damn thing to say. No poems, no prose, no words.

Jesus, I wondered, what do you do with pain so bad it has no redeeming value? It cannot even be alchemized into art, into words, into something you can chalk up to an interesting experience because the pain itself, its intensity, is so great that it has woven itself into your system so deeply that there is no way to objectify it or push it outside or find its beauty within. That is the pain I'm feeling now. It's so bad, it's useless. The only lesson I will ever derive from this pain is how bad pain can be.

One day, after much hemming and hawing, I had decided to see the movie *Ironweed* with my friend Dinah. I was on my way out when the phone rang. My mother was calling from work to tell me that she'd figured it all out, which is how she knew that I should take the semester off from school, return to Cambridge, and just go to therapy every day, devote myself full-time to recovery.

This wouldn't have been such a terrible idea, except that I had already considered checking into a mental hospital and had discarded the idea after Dr. Sterling and a couple of other psychiatrists I consulted insisted that it wouldn't be necessary. Stillman would be completely adequate in an emergency situation, and Dr. Sterling strongly believed in the value of sticking with a workaday routine, of taking classes and swallowing drugs and attending therapy sessions all at once. She believed I had a better shot at learning how to deal with the world while I was still a part of it, and to take time off from school, to sever my connection with Harvard, would deprive me of the many resources—Stillman, for instance—that she thought would be helpful.

Returning to school was the path of least resistance, and Dr. Sterling had convinced me that was my best option. After several fruitful conversations with her, I had even settled it in my mind that somehow, some way, with Dr. Sterling's guidance, I would eventually be *okay*. I would survive breaking up with Rafe and I would survive depression. I didn't completely believe this, but I'd told myself that getting back to school would be the initial step toward any kind of hope. At a point when it was almost impossible for me to make any decisions and stand by them, I'd at least done that much. And now my mother was calling to tell me that as far as she could tell I was so incurably insane that I ought to take time off from school—in fact, she thought I should maybe drop out altogether and work for a living—so that I could maybe get better.

"I've never seen anyone like this," she kept saying.

"Mom, listen, the last thing I should be doing right now is trying to give you perspective, because I'm lacking it myself," I began. "But for Christ's sake, I just broke up with my boyfriend, I've been upset and hysterical, but I'm going to get better. I don't think that your calling me and telling me that I'm in worse shape than even I know is very productive. Because, Mom, I know I *couldn't* be any worse off than I think I am."

"It's just—" she hesitated. "It's just all so crazy. You go running to Dallas and Minneapolis to make yourself feel better and you keep getting worse and worse, and, Ellie, you know I can't cope with this. It's too much for me. I don't understand why you get this way, I don't know what's happening to you, but I want it fixed. Every time you come home, it throws my life into a frenzy because I can't cope with what you're going through, so I want you to go back to Cambridge, and get some sort of job, and go to therapy and get better once and for all."

Her tone combined hysterical fear with mournful horror. Once again, I felt like my depression was a broken car and she was ordering me to *just fucking fix it*, as if my mind could be rewired like a faulty transmission or unresponsive brakes. My mother wanted results, and fast, which is exactly what I wanted, but it didn't seem to work that way. I began to cry because I couldn't understand what my mother thought she would accomplish by saying these things to me. *I* was the one depressed, and somehow she managed to make it sound like I was supposed to feel sorry for *her*. I hated the way our emotional states were still so symbiotic, our moods so mutually dependent. Talking to her for a few minutes had sent me from a cautious belief that I might recover to a feeling that I was cursed, marked like Cain with depression for life. I desperately wanted to get off the phone and wash my hands, my face, my whole body, clean myself of this sullying substance that seemed to spread over me as I listened to my mother.

"Mom," I said, "Mom, I was beginning to resolve to get better, and now you're making me feel like I'm much sicker than I am. Mom, I've got to meet Dinah for a movie, but before I hang up I really want you to tell me that you have faith in me, that you believe I'll be okay. I can't stand this feeling of thinking that you maybe know more than I do, that maybe you're right, that maybe I'm a hopeless case. I can't stand this feeling!" I was practically screaming. "Mommy, please tell me you're with me on this."

"Ellie, I don't know."

I started to contemplate leaving school. One word went through my head: *derailed.* Completely derailed. Thrown off the track of life. It was the same sensation I had when I thought of staying in Dallas at the end of the summer instead of returning to school. I felt like I'd just be somewhere *out there*, that without Harvard to anchor me I'd begin to disintegrate and float into the ozone layer, that years would go by and no one would even know I was gone. It was bad enough to be depressed *and* at Harvard, to be depressed and nowhere at all was implausible. Contrary to everything I'd learned while I'd been there, I still thought of Harvard as salvation.

It took forty-five minutes on the phone with Dr. Sterling for her to convince me that my mother was being impulsive, that everything my mother said was not the word of God. "To be completely frank, Elizabeth," she said, "both of your parents, in my dealings with them, have been pretty crazy. I wouldn't take what she just said too seriously. It sounds like she was having one of her tirades."

I arrived at *Ironweed* an hour late and walked out five minutes later because it was too depressing. *There* was a movie that never should have been made. I didn't want to go home because I was scared to be alone, I didn't want to stay in the theater because I was afraid of the dark, I didn't want to be with my mother because I was scared of her. So I went to an old friend's house, and as soon as I got there I realized that I couldn't bear to be with people, that I really wanted to be alone. As soon as I was out in the street, I realized I didn't want to be alone after all, realized I didn't want to be anything at all.

Tolstoy is frequently quoted as saying something about how all happy families are the same, but unhappy families are all unhappy in different ways. Of course, he's got it totally wrong, completely ass-backward. Happiness is infinite in its variety, and happy people, happy families, can find their joy in so many different ways. It's true that happiness is not very profound as far as art is concerned—it is not the stuff that lengthy Russian novels are made of—but a family that is happy has the ability to do so much, to try so much, to be so much in ways that unhappy families are too smothered in their own sorrow and melodrama to explore. When you're happy, there's so much you can do, but when you're sad, all you can do is sit around and be miserable, paralyzed by despair.

And all the unhappy families are all pretty much the same. All types of misery are identical at the core, which is why for so many years people would tell me to go to AA meetings. They'd say that all addictions are alike, and my addiction to depression or stress involved the same mental mechanism as someone else's alcoholism. In any fucked-up family, whether the problem is that the mother drinks or the father beats the children or the parents want to kill each other, the skeleton of the story line is always the same. The description of what causes the pathology is the same. It's always something about not being loved enough as a child, or being neglected at some other point. Listen to any unhappy person tell his tale of woe, and it sounds like every other tale of woe.

At most, there are two kinds of dysfunctional families: those who don't talk enough and those who talk too much. The former always comes across as the more tragic, the more Eugene O'Neill-ish. These are the families in which everyone is so fearful of expressing not just their emotions, but absolutely anything, that they all drink or do drugs and get fucked up in their silence. Then one day, one of the kids gets busted at school for smoking a joint in the stairwell, or maybe the daughter turns into an anorexic, and the parents see that all kinds of hell is going on while they sip their martinis and suck on their green olives, and finally the whole family ends up seeing a counselor. Pretty soon, they discover that they have trouble communicating, and everyone learns to open up, like it's some great revelation, and the idea that this is any sort of solution to any problem completely baffles those of us from families in which everybody talks too damn much.

One of the terrible fallacies of contemporary psychotherapy is that if people would just say how they felt, a lot of problems could be solved. As it happens, I come from a family where no one ever hesitates to vent whatever petty grievances she might have, and it's like living in a war zone. I am often amazed at the things my mother has no qualms about saying to me. It's not just that she's rather impulsive about expressing her unreconsidered opinions about my mental health, but even trivial matters are fair game. For instance, I'll walk into her apartment and she'll just blurt out, Those shoes are so ugly! And I never asked her. And I like my shoes. And her comment does nothing but make me feel bad. But that's how it is. Her mother does it, her cousins, aunts, everybody. The concept of Who asked you? does not exist in my family, because the concept of individuals doesn't exist. We're all meshed together, all a reflection of one another, as if we were a pot of stew in which all the ingredients affect the flavor.

And I think about my mother and me, and about the way unconditional love has been absent from my life. Not that she doesn't always love me in her heart. But I know that if I'm not being the person she wants me to be, if I'm not the girl who got into Harvard and wins writing awards—if I'm, say unemployed, broke, depressed, and desperate, she just doesn't love me the same way. She doesn't want to know about it. She doesn't want to know if I have sex or if I have a tattoo. She wants only the girl she wants.

Some friends don't understand this. They don't understand how desperate I am to have someone say, I love you and I support you just the way you are because you're wonderful just the way you are. They don't understand that I can't remember anyone ever saying that to me. I am so demanding and difficult for my boyfriends because I want to crumble and fall apart before them so that they will love me even though I am no fun, lying in bed, crying all the time, not moving. Depression is all about If you loved me you would. *As in* If you loved me you would stop doing your schoolwork, stop going out drinking with your friends on a Saturday night, stop accepting starring roles in theater productions, and stop doing everything besides sitting here by my side and passing me Kleenex and aspirin while I lie and creak and cry and drown myself and you in my misery.

Sometimes I think part of the problem relates to ethnicity. We Jews do not have a concept of unconditional love. The God of the Old Testament is judgmental, jealous and vengeful. He gets mad and He gets even. The notion of turning the other cheek, the idea that faith is more important than deeds, these are distinctly Christian concepts. Some say that the difference between Catholic guilt and Jewish guilt is that the former emanates from the knowledge that we are all born already fallen, that there is nothing we can ever do to overcome the original sin; the latter springs from a sense that every one of us was created in God's image and has the potential for perfection. So Catholic guilt is about impossibility, while Jewish guilt is about an abundance of possibility.

I think of my own possibility. I think of the way it is wasted. The way it will always be wasted because I'm sitting here waiting for someone to love me as is.

I don't know why, but when I got back to school I really didn't want to go to Stillman. I think I was sick of all the cranberry juice. But I couldn't sit still in my own apartment with my grief. Everything I'd read about depression and re-covery had stressed that the only way to solve a problem is to go through it, to sit with the feelings, to calm those fight-or-flight adrenaline instincts and just let the pain run its course. Well, fuck that.

I couldn't bear it. I have never wanted out of my skin so badly. Constant suicide thoughts. Total fear. But I didn't want to go to Stillman, and since I had started describing exactly what method I would employ to kill myself—I'd ordered pamphlets from the Hemlock Society, and I was beginning to bone up on what combinations of drugs actually, really, and truly did you in—Dr. Sterling was talking about sending me off to McLean. Which I really didn't want. Don't ask why. At that point, it would have done me good.

But instead of going to a mental institution, I decided to go to California.

Once I got to my cousin's house in Los Angeles, I sat in the sun and soaked in the hot tub. I actually did things like read Sartre in front of the Pacific Ocean. When I realized that Camus's *L'Étranger* begins on a beach, I read that too. I ate frozen yogurt at a combination bookstore and outdoor café in Venice. I risked life and limb crossing a six lane highway to get to a restaurant called the Cheesecake Factory, because for some reason I thought they'd have oysters on the half shell there (they didn't *and* there was a thirty-five-minute wait for a table). I thought about Rafe. I talked about Rafe. I talked to Rafe when I could actually reach him since I was afraid to leave a message.

I worried about finding a summer job, as I'd already been rejected by the *Chicago Tribune*. I interviewed Joni Mitchell for the *Dallas Morning News*. I considered taking the term off from school to write a whole book about Joni Mitchell. I spent more time on the telephone with potential employers in New Orleans and Atlanta and even New York than I did in the California-dreamin' sun. My cousin kept telling me I was too compulsive, that I should relax. She said, You're supposed to be on vacation. She said, You're behaving like one of those studio execs who bring their cellular phones to St. Barts and can't take a day off from the art of the deal. She said, You're too young to be this obsessive and ambitious and feverish.

She didn't seem to see that I was afraid that if I let life take over, if I flowed into my circumstances like some West Coast Zen surfer, I was certain that I would land in a depression and a bog even worse than the one I'd mucked my way into by scrambling around and pursuing this and that, scratching and clawing through these confining tubes of no-options like a hamster in a Habitrail.

Still, she said: Relax, Elizabeth!

And I said, I wish. And I thought about Rafe.

Mostly I thought: It's better in the sun. Everything really does feel better when you wake up to light flooding through the window. It makes it harder to imagine the film of blackness that I could see wrapped around everything in Cambridge and New York in the cold and in the dark. I remembered that Leo, my astrological sign, is the sun ruler, and I wondered how I could make my life more solar. Because by the time I left California, nothing seemed to matter much at all, as if the sun had stroked my brain and fried it to fritters. And I thought: Who needs Rafe?

And then I got back to Cambridge and I needed him all over again and I didn't think I could stand the pain for another minute, another hour, another day. And I remembered how, during winter break, I couldn't stand the pain of missing Rafe for four weeks. Now it was so much worse because the time was not finite. Forever and ever I would be without Rafe because I'd lost him for good.

More Mellaril, and still more pain.

Back to listening to Bob Dylan, back to hearing that cranky, desperate voice sing the most heartbreaking lines I'd ever heard. "If You See Her, Say Hello," "Mama, You Been on My Mind," "I Threw It All Away," "Ballad in Plain D." Why hadn't K-Tel long ago released a compilation called something like *Depressing Dylan Songs for the Broken-hearted?* And then, over and over again, I would listen to all three available versions of "You're a Big Girl Now"—the original *Blood on the Tracks* recording, the alternate take on *Biograph*, and, scariest of all, the live rendition on *Hard Rain*—as if repeated listenings would deflate the song's meaning, make its disastrous lyrics more mundane. But the sorrow and terror of certain works of art—of Picasso's *Guernica*, of Billie Holiday singing "Good Morning Heartache" at the 1957 Monterey Jazz Festival, Sylvia Plath's poem "Tulips," Fellini's *La Strada*—never seem mitigated by exposure. Their power is amplified with every new viewing or hearing or reading, and I just find new elements of tragedy to focus on, new reasons to be empathic. This is especially true of every Bob Dylan song that has ever touched me. There are people who hate his voice, who think he's too nasal and can't sing, would rather hear his work performed by the Byrds or Ricky Nelson or the O'Jays, but they don't understand that for real Dylan fans, the sound of his ragged, edgy vocal cords is the sound of redemption. I wanted to make a whole tape that would play all his different recordings of "You're a Big Girl Now" continuously. This big girl is so very small and fragile after all.

I often didn't even have the energy to get to therapy sessions, so Dr. Sterling would have to talk to me by phone. I didn't have the energy to eat and, strange as this may sound, I didn't have the energy to sleep. All I could manage was lying in my bed. Sometimes, if I couldn't bring myself to get up and refill the glass of water, I would swallow my Mellaril straight and hope it would still metabolize on an empty stomach.

On a Sunday morning, when she didn't have to go to

work or to classes, Samantha got me out of bed by insisting
that the sun was shining on the living room and I would feel
much better on the couch than in my dark room. The conversation we were going to have would inevitably be pointless
because Samantha would always wonder why I couldn't look
at my situation more philosophically, why I couldn't be glad
that I had experienced love with Rafe and take that as a sign
that it would happen again sometime, somewhere, with
someone else. And she pattered away like Pollyanna until I
finally screamed: *Samantha, goddamnit, don't you see I'm desperate! What the fuck do I care how this will seem in ten years, or
ten months. I'm going out of my mind right here, right now, and I
don't think I can bear another minute.*

As usual, I started to cry and Samantha got frenzied, digging her Filofax out of her pocketbook, looking for numbers
or names of anybody who might help me, mentioning a rabbi
in New York or a social worker in Cambridge or suggesting
that I call her father, a psychoanalyst in Washington.

And I just looked at her. "I need a cure," I said. "I know
that I promised myself that getting rid of Rafe would be the
best thing for me because it would help me confront the issues
that his presence shielded me from. But I actually think that
in truth he brought stuff more to the fore."

She nods.

"I know I vowed to be in therapy and get through life
day by day because this is how I'll get better, and in a few
months I'll be stronger because I'll have gotten to the root of
the problem and all that."

More nods.

"But"—I burst into tears—"I don't think I can make it!
I need some protection. I don't see a light at the end of this
particular tunnel right now, and I'm having trouble visual-
izing world peace or inner peace or any of that shit, and I
want to cheat on this plan to go through all this pain right

262 / PROZAC NATION

now. If I were an alcoholic, I'd be saying I want a drink, but since I'm me I don't know what it is I want. But I want it *right now!*"

Samantha says something about understanding how I feel, but I'm barely listening because all I want to do is come up with a way to get blasted off this planet until the pain goes away. I want another trip to California. Or maybe I want a trip to Neptune.

And then suddenly I remember that Samantha's Argentinian ex-boyfriend Manuel lives in London and works in convertible bond sales at a major investment bank. I had managed to have a disquieting fling with Manuel's younger brother when he was a senior and I was a swoony freshman who couldn't believe that his room in Adams House was so big. While Samantha herself was working in London, she lived with Manuel, and by her description he had been very doting and had taken excellent care of her even though she'd cried herself to sleep late at night and walked out in the middle of dinner parties and sobbed on the balcony because she was having her own set of difficulties back then. So I decide that the thing for me to do is go stay with Manuel for a couple of months until I get better.

Samantha smiles at this thought. "I'd love to give Manuel to you," she says. "He's exactly what you need right now." Samantha knows that Manuel is a nice guy who'll buy me dinner and talk to me, which she thinks is a good idea. She also seems to think I'm having a bit of a breakdown here, and the best way to cope is to go with it, preferably while enjoying polite conversation and good meals in fancy restaurants.

Look, he couldn't be any worse for me than Mellaril.

Within a few days and after a few phone calls, the deal is as good as done. Manuel doesn't seem that excited about having me visit—he's heard some pretty weird things about me from his brother—but Samantha is certain that if I am really nice to him, it will all be fine.

I have earned enough frequent flier miles to qualify for a free ticket to London, and I envision liking the city so much that I will decide to get a job and stay. I see London as this wonderful exit from my dysphoric life. I've never been there, never been anywhere in Europe, but I am so excited by the prospect of escaping from the here and now that I figure it will all fall into place once I arrive. I keep thinking that London is the city of Blake and Dickens and all these wonderful writers. I am so desperate to believe that I will like it there that I completely ignore the fact that I hate Blake and Dickens and all those other writers, that I switched from majoring in English to Comparative Literature because I pretty much hate the whole British canon. Byron, Shelley, Wordsworth—the whole bunch of them can go blow as far as I'm concerned. Still, I proceed with my plans, which are all that's keeping me afloat right now, and remind myself that I've always loved those naturey paintings by Gainsborough and Turner, that there are lots of them hanging in the Tate Gallery, that British artists will keep me cheered. I'm doing what I need to do.

Dr. Sterling doesn't know quite what to say about London. She sees me as more scattered and frightened every day, still refusing to go to a hospital but not quite crazy enough to be forceably committed. So she just figures, if London will help, give it a try. It's not exactly that she's given up on me— I know she hasn't, but I think she's waiting for me really and truly to hit rock bottom. She doesn't seem to think I can be helped as much as I need to be until I fall into that desolate place that's nowhere and never. The breakup with Rafe appeared to have strung me to the end of my tether, but I'm still looking for an out, still hoping to escape the brutal sorrow I will have to face before I can get well. She tells me that the therapeutic term for my behavior is *in flight*, and that there's nothing she can do any longer to get me to land properly. I'm going to have to crash on my own.

Luckily, it's early enough in the semester for me to rearrange my whole class schedule to accommodate my travel plans. My tutor, who is also my academic adviser, thinks it would be a really good idea for me to get away for a while, so she's willing to let me read by myself across the Atlantic and turn in my junior essay at the end of the year for full credit. Our tutorial is pass-fail anyway. Another junior faculty member agrees to do an independent study with me on Marx, Freud, and philosophical trends in the late nineteenth century. He feels sorry for me after I tell him my various tales of woe, and he's convinced that if I can get out of the country and still stay in school that would be the best thing. A writing instructor agrees that I can take his course without actually showing up for it, as long as I turn in some stories now and again. I've taken more classes than I needed in previous semesters, so I can afford to take only three now. Harvard's system is pretty thoroughly set up so that a student can be enrolled, even in an honors concentration like Comparative Literature, without taking classes or doing any work. I'm effectively taking time off without actually taking time off, which for some reason assuages my conscience and makes me think I'm less sick than I am.

Only one person bothers to point out the madness of this plan. My sophomore year adviser, who is also the head of my department, tells me I'm making a big mistake. He calls me into his office for a little chat about my academic plans after seeing my application to do an independent study, which he has to approve.

"I know what you went through first semester," Chris says as he smokes and swallows coffee in his office. "I know about the miscarriage—remember, I visited you at Stillman— I know about your emotional problems. But I think you should either really leave school or really get into it. This intermediate approach that you're trying to take is going to lead you down the path of no good. Elizabeth, my advice to someone with your nature—and I think I've gotten to know you pretty well—would be to take some good, challenging courses, really immerse yourself in academics. You love the Bible, you did so well in those graduate seminars you took last year in medieval Hebrew mysticism. Take some more classes like that! Use your mind!" He smiles as he says this, and his optimism kills me. I mean, what mind? I'm loaded on Mellaril. My brain is temporarily out of service. "Go deep into your studies, or else just get out of here for real. Go to Europe and backpack your way around the Continent. Visit Prague, Rome, Berlin, Budapest. Those are wonderful places for a young mind to explore. But don't waste a semester of valuable class time on courses that you don't care about and won't attend to."

As always, I am in tears by the time he finishes with his speech. Of course he's right, but I am completely desperate to both run like hell from Harvard and still, somehow, remain vaguely attached. I know it's precisely this neither-here-nor-there approach that has led me into this marginal existence that is at the heart of my depression, but still I can't stop myself from my behavior. I know, somewhere deep down, that going to London is just more self-destruction, more fleeing from the inevitable, more of an avoidance tactic, but I must persist. "Maybe I really will do all my reading for the independent study and for my tutorial," I say, still crying because I know better. "Maybe I really will get something out of it."

"Oh, Elizabeth." He sighs. "I visited you in the hospital last semester. I know the condition you're in. You're not going to sit around England reading Marx—"

"Yes I am," I interrupt. "I'm going to read in the British

Museum in the very room where he actually wrote *Das Kapital*."

"Oh, Elizabeth." He breathes in deeply. Chris is a scruffy guy, a standard rendition of the groovy academic, always wearing jeans and a tweed jacket with suede patches on the elbows, always smoking unfiltered Camels, always trying to be both friend and wise elder to his students. I actually think that Chris really cares about me as much as any professor at Harvard ever had, though it is hard for me to relate to his discipline of choice, narratology, another sad attempt to turn literature into a science. Still, Chris has always been on my side, and I can tell he is truly struggling with whether to let me get away with this correspondence-course approach to my education.

"I'm not going to keep you from doing what you need to do, and I will sign this independent study form for you because I never want you to be able to say that I stood in the way of your doing something that might possibly be valuable to both your mental and intellectual health," Chris finally says, after a few minutes of brooding and smoking while I sat there weeping and wailing. "But let me just say, I feel certain that this is very wrong. Very, very wrong."

12

The Accidental Blowjob

* * *

now it's raining it's pouring
the old man is snoring
now i lay me down to sleep
i hear the sirens in the street
all my dreams are made of chrome
i have no way to get back home
i'd rather die before I wake
like marilyn monroe
and throw my dreams out in
the street and the
rain make 'em grow

TOM WAITS
"A Sweet Little Bullet
from a Pretty Blue Gun"

A few weeks before I leave for London, I call Rafe and tell him I have something very important to report. In portentous tones, I say that I am going to England and that I am never coming back, as if the idea that I will be lost to him for good might feel like something besides relief. He mutters something or other to me, the kind of thing you say if you are an R.A. in a dorm, something about getting away and gaining perspective, and finally he mentions that it would be a shame to go to Europe and not spend any time on the Continent. I have no idea what he means by this and then he tells me that the Continent is Europe without the British Isles, and it seems stupid for me to try to explain that I have no energy for Paris and Amsterdam and Venice, that I will most likely spend my time in London completely catatonic. If he doesn't know me well enough to know this on his own, he probably doesn't

know me at all and our love was even more of a mirage than
I knew.

On a Saturday night in March, at the Continental Airlines
gate in Newark, my mother, who must feel really bad for me,
gives me $500 in cash to get me "started on a new life." As
if we were in Russia in 1902 and I was off to begin afresh in
the New World, where the streets would be paved with gold.
I wonder how long we can carry on this charade, how long
both of us will be able to perpetuate this fiction that I am
going to London to live? Clearly, if I have any purpose at all,
I am going to London to die or at least to ride out this wave
of death.

I've gotten ahold of a student work visa, I've brought
along a list of phone numbers so long it could rival London's
version of 411 , but somewhere underneath this veneer of
possibility I know that nothing about London will be any
better than anywhere else. My tutor, at the eleventh hour,
had advised me to go to some Caribbean island or even to
Florida—she kept saying that a mood like mine needs Bar-
bados, not Britain—but by then it was too late. Besides, I had
to go somewhere with the premise of actually accomplishing
something other than getting baked on the beach. As I prepared to go to London, I packed a whole bag full of nothing
but reading material—Freud's *Totem and Taboo,* Heidegger's
Being and Time, Milan Kundera's *The Book of Laughter and
Forgetting,* Derrida's *Margins of Philosophy*, a Marx-Engels anthology, and other beach-blanket books like that—because I
was hell-bent on some version of productivity. But somewhere in the back of my mind I must have known better.
How else to explain my last-minute decision to bring Carrie
Fisher's *Postcards from the Edge* along too?

About a week before leaving for London, I'd gone to a
wedding and met Barnaby Spring, a recent Harvard graduate

who lived in Sloane Square and was squandering away his inheritance on various adventures in filmmaking. He'd spent the last year shooting footage in Kenya or Mozambique or Borneo or someplace like that. Barnaby was a London native, a real live Brit, an Eton boy who'd been in boarding school since he was seven years old, and he promised to pick me up at the airport and generally be at my disposal when I arrived. At this wedding, in anticipation of my imminent excursion, I was in a pretty cheerful mood, so I'm sure Barnaby had not the least idea of what he was in for. He might have begun to get a better sense when, the night before I left, I called him six or seven times—this was the first time I'd ever made a call to another continent in my life, so I guess in all the excitement of this novelty I decided to keep doing it over and over again—just to make sure he'd be at the plane, on time, or even a little early. I tried to explain, each time I phoned him, that I was sorry to be so anxious and bothersome, but it was after all my first time in Europe, and I kind of had this excessive phobia, dating back to my homesick days at summer camp, about people meeting me at airports and bus depots. I tried to make light of it—*ho ho ho, I'm so silly*—and Barnaby seemed willing enough to play along. But by about the seventh time I called, it was already 5:00 A.M. in England, and the initial charm that Barnaby seemed to find in my last-minute jitters had worn itself down to nothing but an annoying sleep disruption.

Of course, the whole flight to England was nothing but an annoying sleep disruption. I took one hit of Mellaril after another, but in all my anxiety I couldn't rest on the plane. Just my luck, as soon as I arrived at Gatwick, with customs and whatnot to deal with, the medicine began to take effect. Making my way through the airport felt like walking through an ether-filled cavern with weights on. The air, everything, the whole atmosphere seemed so buoyant, so hard to move through. I almost fell asleep in Barnaby's car (a Jaguar, of course), but I felt that would be rude so I made every effort to stay awake and alert. And it was about then that I realized what a desperate mistake coming to London had been: I had not a single friend in the whole city, I'd be at the mercy of strangers with funny accents, and I'd have to put a lot of energy into being charming and pleasant at a time when I was completely unequipped to do anything but zone out. What an idiot I was! I almost asked Barnaby to take me back to Gatwick right away, to put me on a plane home immediately, that this was the hugest mistake ever.

And then I remembered I had nothing to go back to. No classes, no boyfriend, only some friends who were clearly exhausted from all the care I'd extorted from them over the last few months. It was pretty much England or bust. There was no way out.

Since Manuel was not going to be home until later in the evening, Barnaby took me back to his apartment, which was full of black leather furniture and a black stereo system with black speakers on an array of black shelving surrounding a black television set. I don't know what I expected—something archetypally Anglican, I guess: overstuffed sofas, gold-leaf detailing, Victorian and Edwardian and Jacobean and Elizabethan touches throughout. I was envisioning something out of *Brideshead Revisited,* and instead the place was more like Mickey Rourke's penthouse in *9½ Weeks.* I got this strange feeling, looking around at all the cameras and video equipment, at everything so dark and orderly, that far from being an English gentleman, this guy was more likely to be an amateur pornographer. Or perhaps he was both. After all, there's always been that certain seamy, incest-on-the-manor underbelly to the inbred British aristocracy, all those people in Alistair Crowley's crowd smoking opium, popping laudanum, and fucking their siblings. Barnaby's probably the type who wears bikini briefs instead of boxer shorts, I thought. Leop-ard-skin prints, maybe. And there was something really dis-concerting about how damp and skinny he was—and, well, Jesus, all that black leather.

When I finally realized I was too exhausted to do any-thing else, I asked Barnaby if he'd mind if I took a nap, and then I went into his bedroom and discovered that he had a black leather bed. *Good grief*, I thought. *What am I doing here?*

When I woke up, Barnaby offered me some orange juice, and while I sat on his couch trying to stay awake even though I'd taken about three times my normal dose of Mellaril—and, believe me, I was thinking about taking some more—he sat down beside me, turned my face around, and gave me some version of a kiss. More like he gagged me with his tongue.

"Barnaby," I said nervously, "Barnaby, I guess you don't know that I'm kind of a wreck. I mean, um, I'm here in London trying to recover from—from a lot of stuff. And, well, I just—I just can't do this kind of thing. I really can't."

"But I picked you up at the airport," he retorted. "I said I'd show you around. I assumed you understood."

"Understood what? I didn't know we had a barter agree-ment here."

The conversation ended there because I was frightened. I was alone in this foreign country, and I needed a friend. Barnaby was the kind of goofy chap just made for platonic relationships. And I couldn't believe that this guy had a com-pletely different agenda. *Look at me*, I wanted to say to him, *I am messed up and totally gross! Why the hell would you or anyone else want to get near me?!* Of course, there are some guys who really will fuck anything. Even me. He had told me about how we could go to Stratford-on-Avon and see Shakespeare, that we could drive to the Lake District and check out Wordsworth's house, that we could visit Oxford and Cambridge. He kept telling me about all the things we would do together as he drove me, in my nearly comatose state, into the city from the airport. But it turned out that all that came with a price.

But the worst thing was that I felt too low to be morally outraged. Instead, I was just grossed out. I would have slept with Barnaby in a second if I thought I could have managed to do so without a clothespin on my nose. I was so scared and lonely I'd have done anything for anybody if it meant he'd be nice to me. But Barnaby was too serpentine, too slimy. I didn't want him to touch me.

"Why don't you take me to Manuel's now," I suggested.

"Suit yourself," he said.

Manuel lives in a house in Knightsbridge, the section of London where Harrods is located. The only other people who live around there are investment banker- and management consultant-types who are hardly ever home and have no reason to notice that they live in extremely tight quarters. Manuel and his roommate actually have a whole house to themselves, but it's squashed, tiny and thin, as if a perfectly normal home had been run over and left as flat as roadkill. Upon my arrival, Manuel assigns me—and *assign* is the right word because Manuel is as cold as the drizzle of rain outside— to a little room in the basement that is completely taken up with an ironing board and a lumpy little bed. The only light source is a tiny reading lamp, and there are no windows or ventilation. The mattress feels like it's made out of broken pieces of pottery. I immediately worry that we might reenact "The Princess and the Pea."

But I don't really care about all that—I don't need luxurious accommodations, and living in the dungeon seems an appropriate match for my mood. What's got me worried is that Manuel is actually being mean. It's clear that he doesn't want me here. Before I've even had a chance to fill a glass of water and take another Mellaril he's explaining that this is a favor to Samantha, who he doesn't owe any favors to because she left him in the most heinous way possible (she ran off to the Lake District with another man while he was visiting a sick relative in Italy). It's okay if I stay there and read or do whatever I need to do, but he's busy, he has a life of his own, and it doesn't have any room for me in it.

Whatever happened to polite conversation over good meals at fancy restaurants?

All right, I think to myself, I will live in this dark room with no windows for as long as it takes to get better. I will accept that the only scenery in this little hovel is a pipe across the ceiling and an antiquated iron and pressing board with a pile of trousers next to it, waiting for the laundress. I accept this. I accept that this is my fate. I have come to London to see the absolute bottom, and sure enough, I will.

I sleep fitfully, I can't get out of bed in the morning or even the afternoon, and I think, This is scary. I've got to go home. Even if such a place doesn't really exist.

After I drag myself out of bed that first evening, I spend the next several hours on the phone. I've gone from not knowing how to dial the international operator to becoming something of an expert. I leave messages everywhere because no one's home, it's the middle of the day back in America, where I belong. Finally Samantha calls back. I tell her Manuel will barely even speak to me, it seems I remind him of their breakup, and I can't stay in London another minute. She says stuff like, Oh, poor baby. She says, Can't you just go for a walk and try to take in the beauty of the city? What about that idea about going to read at the British Museum? And don't you at least want to see the Crown Jewels?

When I don't answer, she promises to talk to Manuel.

I call my mother, tell her it's awful here, it's been raining since I arrived, all it ever does is rain. All the rain is falling down all over me, even though I'm indoors. I don't know where to get myself some food, I haven't eaten since I arrived. I think I'm losing my mind.

Come home now, she says. Let's cut our losses. You try one thing after another, nothing works, I'm losing patience with this, I'm tired of getting phone calls from you wherever you are, always in trouble, just come home.

And because she's so adamant, I naturally panic and take the opposite tack. You don't think that might be a little bit hasty? I ask.

Oh, Ellie, she says. Oh, Ellie, I don't know what you should do, but I think—I don't know what to think. This is driving me crazy. You should probably try to give it a few more days, but I don't know. I mean, if you know you're miserable, leave.

My mother starts crying to me from across the Atlantic Ocean, and says she doesn't know what to tell me anymore, why don't I talk to Dr. Sterling. I try to get Dr. Sterling, but she's missing in action. I must leave her twenty messages in a two-hour period, each one getting a step steeper into deep desperation, but I don't hear back from her.

When Manuel gets home from work, I am still in my flannel nightshirt, I am all puffy, there are dots of Clearasil crusted all over my face, I must look like a teenager or even a little girl, which seems to provoke a moment of compassion. "Elizabeth, Samantha called and we talked," he says in his Argentine-gentry accent. "Tell me, what do you want me to do for you? I really can't save your soul, so tell me what the next best thing is."

I have a feeling that it's about that time of day when I'm supposed to start crying to elicit some pity, but I'm on so much Mellaril that my tear ducts are clogged. I scrunch up on the couch, my face contorts, and my voice squeaks in the manner of someone who's about to have a heavy sob, but the tears don't come. It's as if I'm all dried up after all this time. "Maybe," I whimper, "I should go home."

"Samantha said you were thinking that," he says. "Look, that's totally crazy. You just got here. Samantha says you've barely even been out of the United States before, so as long as you're stuck here—if that is how you choose to look at it—you might as well take some of this country in. There are great museums, there is wonderful theater, there is so much to do. And of course, you can easily take a boat or a train to Paris or Amsterdam." As an afterthought he adds, "How can you leave London without at least seeing the Crown Jewels?"

Good God, I think. *What on earth is so great about the fucking Crown Jewels?*

"Oh, Manuel, I know all this seems crazy to you, but—" But what? "But, see, I am crazy right now. I wish you weren't seeing me this way because I'm really not like this." My next line, I think, is something like, *I coulda been a contender.*

He says he understands, he promises to take me to dinner some time later in the week, and in the meantime he recommends that I meet a friend of his who lives nearby and can show me around. His small kindness touches me so much, so disproportionately much, that I am almost okay. I decide that I should bathe, dress, and go to the pub down the street for some food. So I dig up some towels, and find my shampoo and conditioner, think with anticipation and delight about the wonderful vernal scent, practically salivate over the idea of lather and bubbles, and climb a couple of flights up to the master bathroom. But as soon as I walk in, I discover that the windows are open, making the place drafty and horrible. There are not many showers in London, only baths and various extension tubes, which would be fine except that my hair is too long to wash under the faucet. Holding the showerhead in one hand and balancing shampoo in the other seems too complicated, like so much trouble, such a tangle of tasks, that I start to cry, I cry and cry, all because I'm having trouble getting my hair rinsed.

With soap half on and half off, I fall into a towel on the bathroom floor and don't move, except in the convulsive fits of tears, tears so strong they are tougher than Mellaril. The tears go on for hours. Manuel manages to go out to some engagement and come back home, and still, there I am, collapsed on the bathroom floor, a terry-cloth rag doll. He picks me up, carries me into his room, and tries to get me to talk to him, but I'm too scared to say anything. We are both sitting on his bed, he is hugging me, albeit cautiously, because I'm a girl with no clothes on wrapped in a towel. But I am still me, still a sick, sodden mess.

And then, as if this were a very warped version of that old Crystals song, he kissed me.

"So let me get this straight," Dr. Sterling says, when we finally talk, sometime late that night, which is still early evening in Cambridge. "I know you say that you're narcoleptic, and that between the time change and Mellaril you were more or less asleep, but I really don't think there's any such thing as an accidental blowjob."

"Well, call Masters and Johnson right now, because I just gave one a few hours ago," I quip, a sad attempt at humor. "I can be their inaugural case."

"I don't know what to say," Dr. Sterling continues, trying to get us back on a serious track. "Basically, you got to London, you were jet-lagged, the first guy you meet makes a pass at you and tells you he'll be nice if you'll be his sex toy. Then you find out you're staying with another guy who basically sees your visit as a way to act out his hateful feelings toward his ex-girlfriend, who, not knowing he felt this way, sent you there anyway. Plus you're living in a room that's tiny, dark, and uncomfortable, 'like a dungeon.' Then the guy who's being mean to you shows you a little bit of humanity, and you're so grateful because you're one of these people who would always prefer to look for water in the desert even if there's a sparkling spring right down the block, so you end up committing a sexual act that you seem to have had no intention of committing." She sighs. "Plus, you haven't eaten and it's raining. And you're wondering why you're miserable. Elizabeth, anybody would be miserable in a less precarious emotional state than you're already in."

"So you think I should come back?"

"I think you should do what you want."

"I don't know what I want."

"You'll come back when you're ready."

The next day, I forced myself to meet Manuel's friend for breakfast, even though it was still the middle of the night for me. I liked the scones and Devon cream and tea we got at the little coffee shop across the street from Harrods, and I gobbled them down along with some Mellaril, as if I hadn't eaten in days, which I hadn't. He told me about fun things to do in London—museums, theater, museums, theater—those words might as well be the British national mantra.

After that I went to the office that's supposed to help American students find jobs. I planned to work my way through the maze of the Underground, to be a real urban dweller who takes public transportation, but it was raining and it was too exhausting, so I hailed a taxi. As soon as I got to the door of the office and realized I would have to climb up a couple of flights of stairs, I knew this was a mistake. Why was I kidding myself, I had to get back to Manuel's, I had to get back into bed, I had to hide from all this.

It was so obvious that I should have taken the next plane home and checked myself in. But somehow, I couldn't quite do it. I didn't think I'd even have enough energy to get myself out of England. Maybe I would go home in a body bag.

Through the weeks, over every rainy London day that passed by like so much water, I tried to tell myself that I could be back in the United States, resting up in a hospital bed and having nurses bring me cranberry juice. But I would always dismiss the thought. I was convinced that it was better to push myself along in this way. Better to walk around cold, fatigued, and frightened, better to hide under the covers, not eating, not sleeping, barely even *being* in Manuel's creepy dungeon. Better to pretend I might take a weekend jaunt to Paris, to the Eiffel Tower and the Louvre, even though I knew that the City of Light would only be bathed in darkness, even though I knew I didn't even have the energy or wherewithal to stand in line to get a visa, or to go from train to boat to train. Better to just keep faking this lifeless life as long as possible. Better this than feeling the pain head-on in the infirmary. Better to experience it indirectly, in fits and starts, here in England.

I'd think this through, and then I'd down another Mellaril. How much Mellaril was I taking? Who knows. In preparation for my journey to England, I had purchased several prescription bottles' worth, so I had a hefty supply with me. Dr. Sterling had explained to me that Mellaril was only toxic at really high levels. It interacted with the brain, not the heart the way Valium did, so it was a hard drug to OD on. (Presumably, it takes a lot more medication to shut down your brain than it does to slow your heart to a deadly standstill.) That's why it was a good thing to give to suicidal depressives. Even so, lethal or not, I doubt she meant for me to be swallowing these little orange pills every few minutes. But that's pretty much what happens to people who take any kind of medicine for anxiety: When a crisis comes on, they swallow one pill after another, in search of relief. Pop them like M & M's. On the bottle, it says, "Take three times a day, or as needed." *As needed?* Who do they think they're dealing with? *As needed*, in my case, means a pretty constant flow, a portable intravenous dripping into my arm—or, at the very least, new pills digesting in my stomach and entering my bloodstream at all times.

What would it take to make me go back home? Food poisoning should have done it. I caught a nasty case by eating some quiche in the cafeteria at the Tate Gallery (so much for all the wonderful London museums), and for three days I couldn't get out of bed except to vomit. Manuel feels so sorry for me that he lets me sleep in his king-size bed, and I am in such a filthy, effluvial condition that he opts to stay in the cellar room rather than lie down anywhere near me.

Now that I am sick and can't move, I am able to relax and reflect for the first time since I've arrived in England, and I experience a mysterious calm. I like the feeling of not running, the reprieve from life that I'd come to London to find. All the space on this big mattress, the ability to stretch my legs a bit across the serene coldness of these bare white sheets, has become my idea of a good time these days. At this point, even Manuel, seeing that I'm not even physically—never mind emotionally—fit for the leisurely rigors of traveling, is strongly urging me to go home. But somehow, I can't seem to make plans to leave, though I call Continental several times a day to move my departure date around. The computer records every one of these changes, and finally one of the operators, in her mild British manner, suggests that I simply call once when I finalize my itinerary.

As I struggle to make these simple arrangements, it astonishes me to recall what clarity of vision I needed in order to plan this trip to London in the first place. I convinced my mother, various professors and advisers at Harvard, Samantha, Dr. Sterling, and a couple of other minor characters that this was a good idea. I had to lobby the forces. Then I had to get a passport, a work visa, a ticket through my frequent flier program—which involved only a bit less paperwork than it takes to, say, do your long-form tax returns, and even then you usually get an accountant to do it for you. But I was able to manage it because I had such a desperate, deliberate goal: I *had* to get the hell out of my life for a little while. When I want to escape, when I *need* to escape, it is amazing what I am able to do, it is shocking what hidden reserves of strength I can find to undertake the task. You would think that this resourcefulness, if husbanded properly, if channeled into something useful, could really make a difference. My God, I could raise a family of six children and hold down a full-time job with all the energy I expend on depression! But now, lying in Manuel's bed, knowing how simple it would have been to pack my bags, go back home, and take that path of least resistance—which is to say, face my depression—I couldn't exert myself even the tiniest bit. The thought of how bad it will feel to be alone with my feelings—or even at a hospital with Dr. Sterling and my feelings—is so unbearable that it makes London seem like a beautiful reward. I feel like an alcoholic or drug addict who will do anything to avoid going to AA or into rehab, anything to postpone that decision to stop the drinking. But what is it that I'm refusing to stop? Being depressed?

I recently read that treatment for depression costs the United States something like $43 billion annually in lost productivity and employee absence. Depression, in other words, is a huge waste of time and money. It's a drain on so many resources, and even something that is supposed to be delightful, like some time spent in London, turns into a disaster. The guilt I felt constantly, not just about all that I wasted in London, but about all that I was missing out on in every part of my life—my Harvard education was mostly devoted to propping up my mental health—was enough to cause a whole depression on its own.

One night, when I first got to London, I met up with Rhoda Koenig, then the book critic for New York magazine, who had moved to this city on the Thames because she liked it so much better than New York. Rhoda and I had been kind of friendly when I was a high school intern at New York, during one of my wonderfully productive swings, but she had absolutely no patience for me when we dined out in London. "I can't stand listening to you," she kept saying. "When I was your age, I saved up my money, I waitressed for months so I could take myself over to Europe. I didn't have a lot to spend so I stayed in youth hostels, which were uncomfortable, but I was so thrilled to be there. I went to museums, I went to galleries, I saw plays, it was wonderful. But all you seem to be able to do is complain that you miss your ex-boyfriend and you can't plug anything in! This is ridiculous!"

And I couldn't argue with Rhoda. I knew she was right. I know how taxing it is to do something even as small and brief as having a meal with a depressive. We are such irritating people, can see the dark side of everything, and our perpetual malcontentedness kind of ruins it for everybody. It's like watching a movie that you think is great, spiritually uplifting, a lot of fun in spite of its faults, and you're with someone who is in film school or is a professional movie critic, who tends to analyze every moment of the picture until the pure joy that you feel just because you do—no need to explain it—is expunged by all his nitpicking and hairsplitting. And this curmudgeon ends up ruining your night, choking your buzz, killing your joy. Well, that's what it's like to be with someone who's depressed. Only it's not just one movie or just one night. It's all the time.

I wanted Rhoda to understand that I knew I wasn't easy to be with. I kept trying to reach her across the table, to get her to see that I was calling out to her from a very desperate place. I tried, but by then I was so diminished I no longer even knew how to elicit people's sympathy, something I had once done with such skill. Instead, Rhoda ended up making some broad conclusions about how spoiled and ungracious my whole generation was. I was so far gone that I didn't even come across as sad any longer. Just obnoxious.

In the end, it was Noah Biddle, my freshman-year boyfriend of sorts—well, at any rate, he taught me how to do a bong hit—who convinced me to stay in London. He said he'd come for spring break, that we'd rent a car—a Jaguar, he hoped—and travel all over the beautiful English countryside, and all of that would make me feel so much better. We could keep riding through all the manicured greenery of England, past all the lordly manors and mansions, smoking pot and blasting whatever music I wanted to hear on the tape deck, stopping at Stonehenge and Salisbury Cathedral and Oxford and Cambridge, running away from ourselves together.

Noah had recently resurfaced in my life because he and his girlfriend broke up about the same time Rafe and I split, and misery loves company. Suddenly, in his newly humbled state, Noah was all kinds of interested in me, which seemed ridiculous since I was clearly such a mess. I knew that everything he had to offer was too little and too late for me, but I harbored some small pathetic hope that maybe he would, after all this time, be the one to save me, so I agreed to do England with him.

But naturally, his visit to England was an unmitigated disaster. His first mistake was trying to touch me—and I don't mean fuck me, though that would have been a bad thing too, I just mean touch me at all. By the time he arrived in London, I was virtually tactophobic. I felt so much at the mercy of everyone that the only part of me that seemed inviolate was my body. Of course, if anything, quite the opposite was true: Manuel had succeeded in touching me in whatever manner suited his pleasure; it was my body that was quite vulnerable and my mind that was, in fact, untouchable, unreachable by much of anything human. Still, strange and seemingly super-natural forces invaded my psyche at a constant rate. Moods and feelings of a mostly miserable variety swooped down on me like birds of prey at fierce and unpredictable moments. I felt like such a messy, highly reactive creature that I didn't want people to get near me. I felt radioactive, as carcinogenic as uranium, and it made me deeply suspicious of anyone who'd be fool enough to get in touching distance of this poison girl. So when Noah happened to put his arm around my hip in a manner that felt proprietary (he probably thought it was friendly) the first time he walked through the door of Manuel's house, I started to scream. I went on and on about how I was not his property, how dare he act like he owned me, how dare he put his hands on me without my permission. I had been so solitary in that catacomb of a cellar room that the peculiarities of rote human interaction daunted me: Every little thing was grounds for hysteria.

And from the moment he arrived, Noah was all excited to be in London, not even a little jet-lagged, not even wanting to take a nap before we got on with our day, bristling with energy over the thought of such small attractions as Big Ben and Buckingham Palace. And his upbeat mood, rather than having the contagious effect he'd probably hoped for, made me resist him, made me more defiant in my depression. I hated him for not being depressed. He seemed a fool—everyone who didn't feel like me was a fool. I alone knew the truth about life, knew that it was all a miserable downward spiral that you could either admit to or ignore, but sooner or later we were all going to die.

★ ★ ★

We check into the Savoy because Noah wants to stay in London for a couple of days before we start traveling. I am perilously low on cash—in fact, I'm probably down to zero—which is okay because Noah is loaded, and he wants me here even though I'm so unpleasant. He wants me to stay and pretend we're a couple—Lord knows why, no one is watching—even if it means that I spend a lot of time screaming and yelling and telling him how much he annoys me, and he spends a lot of time asking when I last took a Mellaril.

He thinks that if I keep taking my Mellaril, I will behave. He doesn't understand that it makes me too tired to do any of the touristy things he wants to do, running around with his special four-star guide book that's called something like *London on $2000 a Day*, trying to figure out where all the smart and stylish Sloane Rangers—where *tout-le-monde*, as Noah, in his Continental mode, might put it—are dancing and dining these days. He takes to the role of ugly American so naturally it is alarming. He calls ticket agents and spends untold sums of pounds to get orchestra seats to the latest theatrical productions, even though I assure him that I will fall asleep in the middle of anything, even if it is Maggie Smith who has the lead in *Lettice and Lovage*. We meet strangers in restaurants, and he introduces himself as, "Noah Biddle, Harvard College, Porcellian Club," even though I keep telling him that no one in England knows or cares about any of this stuff. Being *anywhere* with Noah is almost more embarrassing than being with your belching, inappropriate Uncle Al at a restaurant like Lutèce, suffering in silence as he asks the waiter for catsup.

"Noah, you know what's funny about you?" I begin one night, as I try to keep from dozing over a dinner of Dover sole. He shrugs, probably hoping I will offer him a pleasant tidbit of insight and not the usual barbs I toss his way. "It's funny how you act so nouveau riche, you try so hard to impress all these people, but you're from this crusty old American family that's supposed to be above this kind of thing. It's like you're still climbing the ladder even though you're already on top." He smiles, as if this were a compliment. He seems to be inured to the fact that he's here with me, that I am miserable, and in my misery I am determined to make him miserable too. I have no idea how I will survive his lack of irony, or my own, for another two weeks.

The day before we are to pick up our rental car—no Jaguar is available so instead we're getting a BMW—Noah and I go to a bookstore to get a guide to the Lake District. I can't imagine why we're going there, Noah will hate it, it's probably so rural that there'll be no place for him to wear his Armani suit or to spend the money that he is withdrawing from a Merrill Lynch credit card fund, which he could probably keep dipping into for another hundred years and still have the principal left to live on.

As we are flipping through paperbacks in the travel section of the store, Noah pulls out his map of London, and tries to plot a nice walk back to the hotel—maybe past Big Ben and through Hyde Park and Bond Street, he suggests. But it's raining and freezing, like always, and this is no time to take any mode of transportation besides a taxi. I am so tired, I have been taking more and more Mellaril, because easy is getting harder every day, so suddenly I find myself on the floor of the bookstore screaming, "I am on the verge of a nervous breakdown here, and you want to walk past Big Ben!"

I keep yelling, pounding my hands on the floor—I am too exhausted to stand up, and in the midst of this tantrum Noah walks away, pretends he doesn't know me. To get even, I start pointing at him from the floor, gesticulating wildly, and say, "That guy is with me, don't let him pretend otherwise! That man is my husband! Don't let him leave without me!"

So Noah explains to the store clerk that I'm having one of my turns, and ushers me out the door, looking mortified.

That night, we are scheduled to go to the theater, and Noah says, Would it be too much to ask you to put on something nice, to make yourself look pretty before we go out on the town? As if this is some society formal. I don't know how to say that we don't know anyone and nobody cares anyway. Still, feeling a little bad about the scene earlier in the day, I put on a black silk skirt and a white silk top with a pearl necklace, and this pleases Noah so much I almost want to change clothes, almost want to put on my ripped jeans and black turtleneck. I've come to resent him so completely for keeping me here in London, for being the one with the money, that I want to do everything I can to annoy him. But the one thing I can't seem to do is get on a goddamn plane and go home. I keep acting like he's imprisoning me when I ought to realize that I'm my own worst jailer.

When we get to Stonehenge the next day, the sun is already setting and Noah thinks it would be really cool to get stoned there while the orange and pink and purple sky shines upon us. Since he let me play Springsteen on the tape deck during the entire drive, I figure I better go along with this. But when we get outside it is windy and cold, and I think to myself, this is *so* high school, the kind of thing you do with some guy who has a customized van that he drives all around the country in pursuit of Grateful Dead concerts and bootleg tapes. But then, how would I know? I never did stuff like this in high school. And I wasn't going to start now.

Later, in Oxford, we meet a couple who end up telling us that they are Jewish and are planning to go to Israel for Passover. I ask them if they will leave a note for me in the Kotel, in the cracks between bricks of the Wailing Wall, because I was always taught that God answers all prayers that are deposited at that hallowed site. All I can think to write, in a childish scrawl on a little piece of paper, is, Dear God, Please send me a miracle that gets me out of this depression because I can't go on this way.

Noah, feeling ecumenical, scribbles something down too. He's probably just asking for a Mercedes for graduation, but maybe I'm wrong.

When we happen to pass through a town called Ipswich, I actually get a bit excited because I figure we can get some Ipswich clams, really fresh and raw, better than the kind they have at the Oyster Bar in Grand Central. So we drive here and we drive there, stopping, asking everyone we see where there's a clam bar, but no one seems to have any idea what we're speaking of, no one has ever eaten a clam. Eventually we realize that it's Ipswich, Massachusetts, where the clams come from. As usual, England has nothing to offer me.

Somewhere on the road, after we've been all over England, after I've cried and ranted and collapsed in Bath and Avon and the Cotswolds and Brighton, as we were heading back to London for a couple of more days before returning home, Noah says to me, "How can you be tired of London? Samuel Johnson said that anyone who is bored with London is bored with life."

"Noah," I answer, "I think you're finally catching on."

As we pull into London, to return to the Savoy before leaving the country, we find ourselves lost in Piccadilly Circus, driving in circles through all the rotaries and one-way streets that make up this central part of the city. This goes on for a while, a half hour at least, and finally I beg Noah to ask someone for directions. I know that men are notorious for refusing to succumb to this simple solution to a simple but rather vexing problem, but still I believe that after all this time Noah will consent to pull over and get help from a passing stranger.

But no. He keeps talking about how finding our way back to the hotel without anyone else's aid will be an adventure, an experience. And this seems so typical of him. I can't imagine what it's like to have a life that is so carefree and easy that the things that most people consider extremely annoying—like getting lost—become some kind of fun diversion. Leave it to Noah in all his ease and luxury to find delight in the annoying. And of course, there is a lot about Noah himself that is very annoying. Aside from all the little tics and mannerisms that perfectly disgust me, Noah could be rightly faulted for just not getting the many nuances in human character. He is, no question, not terribly sensitive or perceptive. But he certainly does know how to travel in style. He even knows how to get lost with real grace. And what, after all, is traveling of any kind except consciously getting lost in the world? Wasn't the whole idea in coming to London that I might just lose enough of myself to find a new, more palatable version? If I can't mellow out and go with the flow of traffic and rain in Piccadilly Circus at a point in my life when there is absolutely nothing at all pressing at me and demanding that I get back to it, then what is there left for me to do?

And I know, know for sure, with an absolute certainty, that this is rock bottom, *this is what the worst possible thing feels like. It is not some grand, wretched emotional breakdown. It is, in fact, so very mundane: Rock bottom is an inability to endure being lost in Piccadilly Circus. Rock bottom is an inability to cope with the commonplace that is so extreme it makes even the grandest and loveliest things unbearable. There is much more to Noah than his refusal to get directions to the Savoy. The guy is an epicure, a man who delights in life, and all he has wanted to do for me in England is share in his good fortune and taste. It is simply amazing to him that all my sorrow cannot be cured by a BMW. And, of course, his inability to calculate how much worse off I am—his inability to understand me or my depression—is a flaw that makes it impossible for me to see his virtues. It is impossible for me to see that what he is doing for me without understanding me is almost kinder than what someone might do who does understand: Noah is giving me his care unconditionally, not because my troubles make sense to him, but because he likes me just the same. His feelings for me are positively parental. He is nice to me because he believes there is something good about me even though all evidence is to the contrary. Everything is paid for, everything is taken care of, we have even had separate beds in most of the charming little inns that we've stayed in along the countryside. Noah is trying to give me this precious gift, this offering of his version of happiness, because that is the best he can do for me. And none of his generosity ever seems nearly as important to me as the fact that, for God-fucking-sake, he refuses to pull over and get instructions when we are lost in Piccadilly Circus.*

Rock bottom is feeling like the only thing that matters in all of life is the one bad moment. Rock bottom is my screaming at Noah, Goddamnit, maybe this is your idea of a good time, but I'm exhausted, I'm depressed, I am only getting out of this country alive because suicide in London would truly be redundant, and if you don't get us some directions, I will strangle you to death!

Rock bottom is everything out of focus. It's a failure of vision, a failure to see the world as it is, to see the good in what it is, and only to wonder why the hell things look the way they do and not— and not some other way. As if there were any way that might look right from behind that depressive fog. It's not as if I hadn't tried to make things work with a man who was nothing like Noah. I mean, Rafe was always overwhelmed with desire to feel my pain with me, he was boyfriend-as-therapist. Still, I felt about as bad with Rafe as I did with Noah, and this sad discovery makes me see what a fresh hell I have landed in. No man is going to solve my problems, no one can rescue me, because I am too sick. Years ago, many many moons ago, back in high school or maybe even earlier, there was a chance that solid love might have penetrated the fumes of my mind and made me feel just a little bit all right. But by the time I got to England, it was too late.

13

Woke Up This Morning Afraid I Was Gonna Live

＊ ＊ ＊

> I know the bottom, she says. I
>   know it with my great tap root:
> It is what you fear.
> I do not fear it: I have been there.
>   SYLVIA PLATH
>   "Elm"

*E*ven under the best of circumstances, it is never pleasant to return home from travel after dark. The estranged familiarity of the place you left behind is so much harder to absorb without light. As I walk in the door of my Cambridge apartment, I get the feeling that the sofa, still covered in white sheets as if at a wake, is going to consume me. The chairs, too, seem predatory. The wildly surreal prints I chose for the living room walls, the Magritte eye and umbrella and hat, all look like demons that might come to life. Without realizing it, I seem to have decorated this place like the set of a film collaboration between Salvador Dali and Luis Buñuel. I keep waiting for the clocks to melt, for the furniture to anthropomorphize. Of course, my own bedroom is eeriest of all, the black leaf curtain I had once found so beautiful now seems just plain funereal.

I am supposed to pack up a bag to take with me to Stillman—toiletries, clothes, necessaries—but what's the point? There's nothing I want, nothing I can use. As far as I can tell, the sweatpants and pajama top I have had on since I got back from England will never be peeled off of my body again. I have to remember to leave a note telling them that this is what I want to wear in my coffin, this is my ten-feet-under attire. Because I'll have no occasion to change my outfit from this day forward: Bathing seems like an exercise in futility, like making my bed or brushing my teeth or combing my hair. Clean the slate, then let it get sullied once more. Wipe it down, and wait for more filth. This inevitable pattern of progress and regress, which is really what life is all about, is too absurd for me to continue. The moment in *The Bell Jar* when Esther Greenwood realizes after thirty days in the same black turtleneck that she never wants to wash her hair again, that the repeated necessity of the act is too much trouble, that she wants to do it once and be done with it, seems like the book's true epiphany. You know you've completely descended into madness when the matter of shampoo has ascended to philosophical heights. So as far as I'm concerned, the last shower I took is the last shower I will ever take.

Whatever remnant of will I once had to get better has slipped away, drowned in the Atlantic Ocean while I flew overhead. For the longest time, my depression seemed wrong, it seemed like an outer appendage, a bothersome spare limb that was tacked onto a life that should have been happy. But I don't believe that anymore. I believe it is right and good that I should be so low. I believe that the nature of life—even normal, sane, not-depressed life—has worn me down, and it will wear me down some more. It is just a fact that if I am to grow up, eventually get married, and have kids, and do all those happy things, along the way I will have so much trial and error to go through, so much living that I can anticipate only with dread. There will be so many more Rafes, so many more heartbreakers, so many more cycles of elation at the first kiss, and devastation when it's over. I accept this pattern of relationships as a perfectly decent way for people to make their way through the mating game—but I can't handle it. I am so wrecked already, so unstable, a piece of work who was never given the tools it takes to deal with what everyone else considers business as usual. I am not equipped with any emotional resilience, can't go with the flow, can't stand steady while the boat rocks and rolls. Once, so long ago, I had it in me, but now it's too late. Years of depression have robbed me of that—well, that *give*, that elasticity that everyone else calls perspective.

And now I don't even want it anymore. I believe there is an integrity to my intolerance: Why does the rest of the world put up with the hypocrisy, the need to put a happy face on sorrow, the need to keep on keeping on? Why is everyone so willing to be so cool when she unexpectedly crashes trays in the dining hall with a person who only the night before saw her naked and vulnerable, who in the light of day is a stranger, a person who nods hello? Why do people put up with all the indignities that are par for the course in their interpersonal affairs, and then, with equal resilience, go about their public lives, spending so much of their time bumping up against a bureaucracy whose whole purpose is to keep telling you *no!*? I don't know the answer. I know only that I can't. I don't want any more of life's vicissitudes, I don't want any more of this try, try again stuff. I just want out. I've had it. I am so tired. I am twenty and I am already exhausted.

The only reason I agree to go to Stillman—besides the fact that a couple of orderlies are scheduled to come here and get me—is that I am too tired to do anything else. It takes energy and will to commit suicide, and I don't have either. Dr. Sterling says she's going to put me on some new drug, but she isn't aware that I've already crossed the line, I've already surrendered to the death urge. *I refuse to get better.* I only hope that whatever pill she gives me makes me feel well enough to plot my own end, to gather the medicines or other methods of destruction in order to make this suicide a success and not just one more wimpy attempt by another hysterical girl who wants help. Because I don't want their fucking help anymore.

I have studiously tried to avoid ever using the word madness *to describe my condition. Now and again, the word slips out, but I hate it.* Madness *is too glamorous a term to convey what happens to most people who are losing their minds. That word is too exciting, too literary, too interesting in its connotations, to convey the boredom, the slowness, the dreariness, the dampness of depression.*

You associate madness with Zelda Fitzgerald in all her rich, gorgeous, cerebral disturbedness, or maybe you think of it as something that members of Aureliano Buendía's family sank into at the incestuous end of One Hundred Years of Solitude. *Madness is something of the fiery hot tempers of Latin America or the Deep South, of Borges and Cortázar or William Faulkner and Tennessee Williams. Madness is delightful to the beholder, scary in its way, but still fun to watch, a sport for spectators and rubberneckers who can't avert their eyes from the awfulness that they know they shouldn't be seeing. Madness is Jim Morrison swinging suggestively out of the seventh-floor window of his suite in the Chateau Marmont; it's Elizabeth Taylor and Richard Burton duking it out through the cramped camera angles of* Who's Afraid of Virginia Woolf?; *it's Edie Sedgwick in all her anemic, anorexic beauty, trying to do herself in with amphetamines and pearls while dancing on the table at Ondine and posing for* Vogue *as a youthquaker; it's Kurt Cobain, in every one of those Nirvana videos, looking like a man who is sick, deeply sick, who needs help badly and wears his desperation like a badge of cool; it's Robert Mitchum, with his tattooed knuckles, preaching and ranting in* The Night of the Hunter; *it's Pete Townshend smashing his perfectly good guitar to bits and pieces; it's every great moment* in rock and roll, and it's probably every great moment in popular culture.

But depression is pure dullness, tedium straight up. Depression is, especially these days, an overused term to be sure, but never one associated with anything wild, anything about dancing all night with a lampshade on your head and then going home and killing yourself. The elegance and beauty and romance of Cio-Cio-San as she bleeds to death in Madame Butterfly, or of the double suicide in Romeo and Juliet: That is the domain of madness alone. The word madness allows its users to celebrate the pain of its sufferers, to forget that underneath all the acting-out and quests for fabulousness and fine poetry, there is a person in huge amounts of dull, ugly agony.

Why must every literary examination of Robert Lowell, of John Berryman, of Anne Sexton, of Jean Stafford, of so many writers and artists, keep perpetuating the notion that their individual pieces of genius were the result of madness? While it may be true that a great deal of art finds its inspirational wellspring in sorrow, let's not kid ourselves about how much time each of those people wasted and lost by being mired in misery. So many productive hours slipped by as paralyzing despair took over. None of these people wrote during depressive episodes. If they were manic-depressives, they worked during hypomania, the productive precursor to a manic phase which allows a peak of creative energy to flow; if they were garden-variety, unipolar depressives, they created during their periods of reprieve. This is not to say that we should deny sadness its rightful place among the muses of poetry and of all art forms, but let's stop calling it madness, let's stop pretending that the feeling itself is interesting. Let's call it depression and admit that it is very bleak. Sure, madness draws crowds, sells tickets, keeps The National Enquirer in business. Yet so many depressives suffer in silence, without anyone knowing, their plight somehow invisible until they adopt the antics of madness which are impossible to ignore. Depression is such an uncharismatic disease, so much the opposite of the lively vibrance that one associates with madness.

Forget about the scant hours in her brief life when Sylvia Plath

*was able to produce the works in Ariel. Forget about that tiny bit of time
and just remember the days that spanned into years when she could not
move, couldn't think straight, could only lie in wait in a hospital bed,
hoping for the relief that electroconvulsive therapy would bring. Don't
think of the striking on-screen picture, the mental movie you create of
the pretty young woman being wheeled on the gurney to get her shock
treatments, and don't think of the psychedelic, photonegative image of
this same woman at the moment she receives that bolt of electricity.
Think, instead, of the girl herself, of the way she must have felt right
then, of the way no amount of great poetry and fascination and fame
could make the pain she felt at that moment worth suffering. Remember
that when you're at the point at which you're doing something as desperate and violent as sticking your head in an oven, it is only because the
life that preceded this act felt even worse. Think about living in depression from moment to moment, and know it is not worth any of the great
art that comes as its by-product.*

The first order of business, when Dr. Sterling comes to see
me at Stillman, is finding a that will work. Clearly, the whole
Mellaril experiment has been something of a failure, perhaps
not a colossal failure, but considering the condition I'm in
and its progression while I've been under the influence of this
exhausting neuroleptic, it might be safe to say that Mellaril is
not for me.

Before I left for England, I had a consultation at the
Affective Disorders Clinic at McLean, and the evaluating
physicians were completely gung ho about a new pill called
fluoxetine hydrochloride, brand name Prozac. They thought
I was the perfect candidate for the drug, and they were all set
to enroll me in a study that would have allowed me free
treatment and medical care. But I was leaving for London,
and besides, Dr. Sterling is a bit more conservative; she
doesn't think that just because something is new or that all
the radical psychopharmacologists at McLean are hyped up

about it means it's the right thing to take. Fluoxetine had been virtually untried beyond the confines of McLean and other similarly progressive meccas of pharmaceutical research and treatment.

Dr. Sterling wants me to know what other drugs are available. Even if she ends up opting for fluoxetine, she thinks it's important that I understand the process she has gone through in making that decision. First, there are the standard tricyclic antidepressants, formulated and introduced in the fifties, drugs like Tofranil, Elavil, and Norpramin, which are, at this point, available quite cheaply in their generic forms as, respectively, imipramine, amitriptyline, and desipramine. These drugs mainly act on the production of norepinephrine and serotonin, two chemicals—scientifically known as neurotransmitters—that the brains of depressives are either lacking or not using efficiently. Essentially, these drugs prevent secreting cells from reabsorbing these neurotransmitters, thus allowing them to circulate and stimulate the next nerve cell into production. Psychiatrists have had a fair amount of luck treating depression with these drugs over the years, but they have some annoying side effects—drowsiness, weight gain, dry mouth, constipation, blurred vision—and have mostly been used by people incapacitated by depression.

Then there are the monoamine oxidase inhibitors (MAOIs) like Nardil and Parnate, another type of antidepressant that works by preventing the breakdown of surplus neurotransmitters, thus creating larger reservoirs within the nerve synapse. The MAOIs work on norepinephrine, serotonin, and dopamine—the most commonly implicated chemicals in mood disorders—but the lack of specificity has its disadvantages. MAOIs require some very rigid dietary restrictions that can be too taxing for a psychologically unstable person to observe. People taking MAOIs can't eat certain cheeses, pickles, vinegar, or drink rich red wines, for instance, a fact that was discovered by doctors only after patients taking the drug consumed these substances and died. (In a famous legal and medical scandal, the lawyer and author Sidney Zion's daughter Libby died in a hospital after a doctor's error had resulted in her taking a dangerous combination of drugs. Nardil was one of the substances believed to have precipitated her death.) With MAOIs, the fear is that a suicidal patient might take advantage of this fatal opportunity to try a comparatively pleasant, and frankly gourmet, method of death, which might only involve chowing down on some Stilton or imbibing a goblet of Chianti.

Then there's Prozac. It is so new at this point that Dr. Sterling still refers to it as fluoxetine. Prozac, like Zoloft, Paxil, and other drugs of its type which were not yet available as I lay in Stillman in 1988, acts only on serotonin. It is very pure in its chemical objectives. Its drug family will come to be known as selective serotonin reuptake inhibitors (SSRIs), and it can act very powerfully and directly within its narrow domain. Since fluoxetine's aims are less scattershot than that of its predecessors, it tends to have fewer side effects.

The McLean people recommend fluoxetine because they have diagnosed me with *atypical depression*. This diagnosis was not easy for them, or for Dr. Sterling, to come by, as the occasional appearance of manic-like episodes (for instance, during my energetic first month in Dallas) might indicate that I suffer from either manic-depressive illness or cyclothymia, a milder type of mood-swing disease. But in the end, the diagnosticians conclude that I've been too persistently down and not florid enough in my manic periods to be bipolar. Atypical depression is long-term and chronic, but the sufferer's mood can occasionally be elevated in response to outside stimulus. This diagnosis seems a better way to explain the periodic occasions when I seemed happy or productive, but would always return to my normally depressed state in perfect boomerang fashion. Apparently—and this is news to me, be-cause I assumed that most depressions went on for years like mine—the natural history of "typical" depression involves a person becoming despondent in response to some situation or turning point in life, then going to therapy, working it through, perhaps taking some drug, and recovering in a cer-tain amount of time. Another typical depression would be much more extreme: A person goes completely nuts, ends up in a mental hospital or attempts suicide, and recovers in time through intensive treatment. But in both scenarios, the symp-toms achieve some sort of apex and logical conclusion.

The atypically depressed are more likely to be the walk-ing wounded, people like me who are quite functional, whose lives proceed almost as usual, except that they're depressed *all* the time, almost constantly embroiled in thoughts of suicide even as they go through their paces. Atypical depression is not just a mild malaise—which is known diagnostically as *dysthymia*—but one that is quite severe and yet still somehow allows an appearance of normalcy because it becomes, over time, a part of life. The trouble is that as the years pass, if untreated, atypical depression gets worse and worse, and its sufferers are likely to commit suicide out of sheer frustration with living a life that is simultaneously productive *and* clouded by constant despair.

It is the cognitive dissonance that is deadly. Because atyp-ical depression doesn't have a peak—or, more accurately, a nadir—like normal depression, because it follows no logical curve but instead accumulates over time, it can drive its victim to dismal despair so suddenly that one might not have both-ered to attend to treatment until the patient has already, and seemingly very abruptly, attempted suicide.

Dr. Sterling, everyone at McLean, and every psychiatrist I've met since has admitted ignorance about why the specif-ically serotonergic action of fluoxetine seems to work for atypical depression in ways that the tricyclics don't. Dr. Sterling could have prescribed something like imipramine for me months ago, but all the case histories seemed to indicate that it would have done no good. Since the MAOIs are highly toxic when mixed with the wrong foods, there was no way Dr. Sterling would administer one of them to me in my precarious state. Besides, the conventional wisdom has always held that the best treatment for atypical depression is therapy alone. But now that fluoxetine is on the market as Prozac, there is a sense that at long last there is a chemical antidote for this disease.

It is interesting what happens to me as I lie in my bed in Stillman and listen to Dr. Sterling explain my diagnosis and my options. Having my situation boiled down to these scientific terms, to a disease I can look up in the American Psychiatric Association manual, gives me some kind of renewed sense of hope. It's not just depression—it's *atypical* depression. Who would have thought they have a name to describe what is happening to me, and one that pinpoints my symptoms so precisely? In the book *Understanding Depression*, Donald F. Klein, M.D., and Paul H. Wender, M.D., characterize atypical depressives as people who "respond positively to good things that happen to them, are able to enjoy simple pleasures like food and sex, and tend to oversleep and overeat. Their depression, which is chronic rather than periodic and which usually dates from adolescence, largely shows itself in lack of energy and interest, lack of initiative, and a great sensitivity to periodic—particularly romantic—rejection." Those sentences perfectly delineate my symptoms. I feel suddenly so much less lonely. For so many years I wondered what was wrong with me, why I felt so awful but still, somehow, didn't completely fall apart. For years I thought there would be no help for me until I got progressively worse, rather like someone who would like to be employed but knows she can't possibly earn as much at a job as she receives from a welfare check, and so flounders deep into poverty in order to receive public assistance.

Dr. Sterling tells me that she has suspected from the start that the cache of feelings and behaviors that characterize atypical depression described my situation exactly. But she's never bothered to mention it because there isn't any reason to draw the symptoms of a depression into a particular category unless a therapist is about to prescribe an antidepressant. Enter Prozac, and suddenly I have a diagnosis. It seems oddly illogical: Rather than defining my disease as a way to lead us to fluoxetine, the invention of this drug has brought us to my disease. Which seems backward, but much less so later on, when I find that this is a typical course of events in psychiatry, that the discovery of a drug to treat, say, schizophrenia, will tend to result in many more patients being diagnosed as schizophrenics. This is strictly Marxian psychopharmacology, where the material—or rather, pharmaceutical—means determine the way an individual's case history is interpreted. But right now, lying in Stillman, I am in no position to do this kind of critical thinking. I am simply reminded of the way I've always felt that the onslaught of my depression occurred gradually and then suddenly—an ostensible paradox, but that's why it's atypical.

Antidepressants, unfortunately, are not fast-acting. They take anywhere from ten days to three weeks to kick in, and sometimes six weeks isn't long enough. So of course, without the Mellaril, my little orange knockout pills, without any sort of life support system, I feel like hell in the beginning of my Prozac days. My roommates have brought me my little Panasonic tape recorder—the same one I used to take to junior high with me to play Foreigner while I hid and cut myself in the locker room—and I scrunch up in the fetal position and listen to Lou Reed over and over again, no longer finding the twisted poetry of Bob Dylan or the lovesick folkie blues of Joni Mitchell even vaguely apposite. *I'm too afraid to use the phone / I'm too afraid to put the lights on.* I listen to the same song, the same words, the same snarly voice repeatedly, like a broken record.

I wonder how long I can lie here, waiting for this fluoxetine stuff to work. But that's the plan, that I'll stay put for however long it takes. I keep thinking of a John Berryman poem in which he talks about lying under a thick green tree, or maybe it's leafless and bare, a weeping willow, waiting for his happy hour. *Minutes I lay awake to hear my joy* is the last line. I guess I'm doing the same thing. Waiting, waiting, waiting. Waiting for Godot. Waiting for the Robert E. Lee.

It's going on a couple of weeks since I last bathed; I am so greasy and broken out that I don't even feel human anymore. I feel more like some piece of poultry, a Perdue chicken going through the forty-four kinds of inspection mentioned in the ads, as an attendant comes in each morning and sticks a needle in my arm to draw some blood and shoves a thermometer in my mouth to take my temperature, as if I were a sick person in the physical sense, as if I were here with pneumonia or mononucleosis or any of the more usual reasons that bring people to Stillman.

Dr. Saltenstahl, the attending physician at Stillman, comes to see me a couple of times a day. I keep telling her I've never felt so low, I can't see any reason to go on like this. And she assures me that someday, when I've worked out a philosophy to live by and found the things that I like to do, I will be happy, I will be fine. She reiterates that the medication I'm on is excellent, has worked wonders for depressed people whom nothing else would help in its pilot programs. She says things like, Give it time.

Dr. Sterling comes to visit me and I keep telling her the

same thing, that the fluoxetine isn't working quickly enough. And she too says, Give it time.

God, do I wish that every psychiatrist I have ever dealt with could know what it's like to be a patient and to feel desperate. I wish they could know what it's like to wake up every morning afraid you're going to live. Dr. Sterling keeps telling me that this drug will start working in a week or two, but she doesn't understand that I don't *have* a week or two. She doesn't understand that the pain is so bad that I don't want to live like this anymore. If Dr. Sterling told me, if she promised me, if she guaranteed me beyond a shadow of a doubt that within ten days the fluoxetine would make me feel completely better, I wouldn't care at all, it would not make a whit of difference: It would not make it worth getting through these days, these hours.

I try to convey this to Dr. Sterling, and though she may truly sympathize, all she can say is, "What can I do to let you know that help is on the way? How can I make you see that you *will* get better?"

"You can't."

She doesn't respond.

"I want shock therapy," I say. "I've read about it recently, and apparently it works quite well on people who are beyond hope. Knocks your brain out a bit. Or else I want morphine. I want something that will work *now*."

Through this whole conversation, I'm lying perfectly still on my side, my hair matted down like a layer of glossy brown paint on my head, my voice slightly muffled because I'm sunk into a pillow. I am speaking in a monotone, and I hear myself as if from a great distance. I know the person that is lying in my bed is so low that she's asking for electroconvulsive therapy, knowing that in all its history shock has been administered to reluctant patients who beg to be spared this procedure, but I'm too detached to find my request odd. Right now I'll do anything to feel better. A frontal lobotomy, even.

"Look," Dr. Sterling says, pushing off the windowsill, where she's been leaning, "I know you're really in pain, but I'm going to have to give this some thought." She gathers her helmet and begins to wheel her bike toward the door. "I am so certain that the fluoxetine is going to help you really soon that I just have to find a way to keep you going through these next few days. It's already been a week, and I actually think you're doing better. You may not see it, but I do. Your *symptoms*, which is to say, what you are feeling, may not have improved, but your *signs*, that is, the way you appear to people who know you well and can judge, are much better."

I look at her, even from my prone and expressionless vantage point, like she is totally crazy. "Look at me," I mumble. "You can't really tell me you think I look better?"

"No, not in obvious ways, but I've been watching you very closely, so that I can see some improvement in you even though you've been in the same position every time I've been here." She scratches her head and pauses to think for a minute. "What I'm going to do is up your dose of fluoxetine to two pills a day, since I think one has gotten a partial, but not total, response. I'm confident that that will work very soon. In the meantime, I actually think you should get out of Stillman. This might be unorthodox, since in your condition you ought to be protected, but I think that lying here, being so isolated, might be making you worse. It seems to be a pattern with you that certain things that were solutions at one point eventually become part of the problem so you have to find new solutions. It's a sunny day. Go outside. That might help."

The next morning, I'm back in my miserable bedroom in my eerie apartment still waiting for the fluoxetine to work, and Samantha bangs on my door and wakes me just after 9:00.

"Elaine from your mother's office is on the phone," Samantha says, as she pushes the door open. "She says it's urgent."

I want to ask Samantha if she can drag the line into my room, which, of course, she can't do because it's not physically possible. Every time I meant to get an extension cord for the phone I was too depressed to go to the hardware store. I want Samantha to make some excuse for me, but I have this feeling I better get up and deal with this. "Hi, Elaine, how are you?" I ask, trying to be pleasant.

"I'm fine, thanks," she begins, "but, Elizabeth, I don't know how to tell you this, but your mother was mugged this morning."

"Oh my God!" Just when I thought life couldn't get any worse. "Did anything serious happen? Is she badly hurt?"

"Well, the guy beat her up pretty badly. She's very bruised. And he broke her arm." The way she's talking, I think there might be some unspeakable detail she's leaving out, but after a minute I realize that that's just Elaine's voice working on my paranoia.

"Is anyone with her? How did this happen?"

"She was walking on Sixty-fifth Street at 6:00 this morning, and this guy just lunged after her," she says. "She called me from the hospital, and I went to see her. We had a cry together, but she seems okay now."

"Jesus, I guess I should come down."

"She said to tell you that she's all right, no need to leave school."

"But now she's all alone, right?"

"Well, the police came by with pictures of suspects."

"And?"

"The guy was wearing a hood, she couldn't see him."

"Oh."

I know I have to get down there, I just don't know when I can. It's Friday. Maybe first thing Saturday morning.

"Elaine, I mean, is she okay?"

"She's badly hurt." Elaine doesn't know what I mean. I mean: *Is she losing her mind? Is anyone visiting her?* I know my mother. She is very solitary. Never remarried, isn't the sort to spend hours on the phone gabbing with her girlfriends, she and her sister haven't been getting along lately, her parents are in geriatric lala-land most of the time, my grandfather wondering if I want purple milk or green milk with my breakfast. I'm pretty much all she has, and I'm falling apart right now.

When I call my mother, she insists that I don't have to come down. But then she starts crying about how he didn't have to knock her over and beat her, that she would have given him her bag without all that. She starts asking me why he kept punching her and kicking her in the face while she lay on the ground, she wants to know why he kept brutalizing her even after he had her pocketbook. And then she says she knows they'll never arrest the guy because she can't identify him and that for the rest of her life every young black man she sees might be the one who did this to her. And I just, I don't know what to say, can't think of a single bullshit comforting thought that can possibly put a redeeming gloss on this incident. Instead I promise that I'll take the first shuttle in the morning.

As I get back into bed, I pray for adrenaline, I beg God to make the fluoxetine suddenly start to work, to endow me with whatever it takes, whatever greatness is contained within the human spirit, that will allow me to rise to this occasion and take care of my mother.

My mother's room at Roosevelt Hospital is large and tiled. It almost looks like a locker room. A meat locker or a mortuary, a place where bodies rot. It's not at all cozy like Stillman. I walk over to her bed, and there she is, this tiny person with her arm in a sling, two black eyes, a completely bruised face. She is colored a range of purples and blues and yellows, and she looks out of place in this bed, as if she were dropped there out of the sky with no landing gear. That's all that keeps running through my head: This room is so large and she is so small, how will anyone ever know that she is here? She has disappeared in the universe, as I've always feared I might do, and it seems like I'm the only person who might be able to find her.

The nurses' aides malinger at their station down the hall from the room. My mother keeps insisting she doesn't want to see anyone besides me, and I wonder how I can keep from obsessing about suicide long enough to do whatever she needs. The other people occupying this large room all seem to be in their own microcosms of pain, letting out groans or grunts every so often that would seem to indicate that they're still alive. They've got purple legs, necks held in place by gadgetry that look like bird cages, faces slashed and restitched, with lines of red blood seeping through the bandages where the seams of skin are held together. This whole Dantesque scene, this whole carnival of the damned, is too close a match with my mood.

"Oh, Mommy," I cry when I finally lean down to kiss her. "Oh, Mommy, what happened to you?" I feel myself gasping the way I would if I were crying, but there are no tears. I rub my eyes instinctively, but they are dry. I wonder if fluoxetine has the same anticholinergic effect as Mellaril, turning off the tear ducts, and I feel so terrible being deprived of my tears at a time like this.

I hug my mother, and she hugs me back weakly, one arm flapping limply on my back like a door with a broken hinge, and she says something like "Hi, sweetheart."

I don't want to hear about what happened, I don't want one more reason to feel unworthy of my misery in the face of someone who has real reasons to feel terrible, but I know

I have to ask. "Mom, are you in terrible pain? Have they given you enough painkillers?" I start to imagine myself momentarily transformed into a valiant person, forced into some heroic scene like Shirley MacLaine in *Terms of Endearment* when she runs out to the nurses, who are indifferently filing their nails, and screams that they *must* give Debra Winger something for her pain *right now*. I imagine myself rising to the occasion.

But it won't be necessary. "Yeah, I'm fine, really I am," my mother says. She's always been a trouper. She doesn't even like having a Demerol intravenous because she's one of those stoic antidrug people who aren't even comfortable taking aspirin for a headache. She's one of those people—bless their souls—who don't complete the Percodan or codeine prescriptions that they get after surgery. Can we possibly be related?

She seems to want to sleep, which is good because I am desperate to get out of there. I feel suffocated and helpless. Here she is, in the worst condition she's ever been in, and all I can think is that I am not strong enough to handle this, I will never get through this. I start wishing I had siblings, I wish my mother had a boyfriend or even a best friend she sees regularly who could come help me out, but the only person she really wants to see is me. I feel like her mountain. Only I'm about to have an avalanche.

My mother is supposed to leave the hospital Sunday morning and my aunt and grandparents are going to come into the City to welcome her home. This is going to be one of those grotesque family rituals, epitomized in the extreme in movie scenes of parents greeting their G.I. son at the airport, trying not to act shocked as he returns from Vietnam a wheelchair-bound paraplegic. And when the boy has to be carried in and out of the car, when he can't move by himself at all, when he even needs to be accompanied to the bathroom like a little kid for God's sake, everyone must smile and be warm and act happy to see the crippled man who was once such a wrangly, handsome lad, who can now do nothing for himself. So they try to smile, but their expressions betray the truth: They are grossed out.

My mother, no surprise, looks like hell when I wheel her out of Roosevelt Hospital. Her face is still bloated and blown, colorful in decorator neutrals—burgundies, khakis, grays. Because she was wearing her pocketbook New York-style—the strap across her chest, instead of just balancing on her shoulder, to protect the bag from pickpockets—the mugger had to pull and twist her quite hard to get the thing off. As a result he broke her arm, and she will need to have microsurgery to repair the shattered bone. In the meantime, some of her nerves have been at least temporarily severed, and her right arm may never be completely functional again. She is a lefty, as luck would have it—or perhaps luck is the wrong word—but it's clear to me that she will be pretty helpless for the next few days. And I feel the wave drowning me.

As I load my mother into a taxi, toting her shopping bag of bloodied clothing, I try to act concerned. Which I guess I am, but really I'm too miserable to care. I feel duty bound, but I am so absorbed in my own depression and misery that I almost hate her for burdening me with this now. In general, there is nothing like a genuine crisis to galvanize a person out of a bad mood, to snap her into a dealing mode. But I am so far gone at this point that the special surge of necessary energy, the adrenaline rush, is not hitting me at all. I am simply plodding along, forcing myself to care at all. I hate myself for being so low and I hate my mother for needing me to be otherwise. And I am on the whole disgusted that I am even thinking about these things at a time like this.

I think about what life must have been like for her before

I was born. She never had a very good relationsip with her parents or sister, she barely had anything much to say or do with my father, so when she had a baby, she must have thought, At last here is someone just for me. Motherhood must be like that. It is probably the only experience that most women ever have of ownership and domination. My mother is as helpless as an infant herself, but I imagine that aside from all the physical pain this must be vaguely blissful for her: For the first time in a long time, circumstances have brought this thing back to her, this thing that is hers and hers alone. And I feel so bad because I am so scared I will not live up to it.

I somehow survive the relatives' visit, although I space out and nod off frequently. My grandmother is courageously try-ing to keep the conversation going in this glum little circle as we sit around eating an improvised lunch in the dining room, and all I keep saying in response to her questions is, I'm sorry, Grandma, what was that? As soon as anyone finishes eating anything, if a plate sits idle for even a few seconds, I grab it and run to the kitchen to wash it. Anything to get away, even for a minute or two. I have never been so eager to clear the table and load the dishwasher as I am that day.

My grandmother keeps asking my mother what's wrong with me, why I seem so tired and gloomy, and I'd overhear my mother saying something like, She's had a hard day. At one point I walk into my bedroom to get something, and I nearly collapse. When I am this depressed, every small activity is a body blow, and I feel knocked out and somnambulent all the time.

Dr. Sterling always tells me that it takes a lot of energy to be depressed and even more energy to get better, and the reason many depressives choose to go to the hospital is that it's the one place where they aren't forced to use their energy on any other activities. I start thinking that as soon as I go back to Cambridge, I'm going to check myself back in, I'm so tired from just trying to stay awake.

When the family finally leaves, I am relieved because I can't deal with them and frightened because I can't deal with myself either. I go into my mom's room to keep her company for *60 Minutes*. "How are you doing, Mom?" I ask, as I sit with her.

"I'm okay," she says. "You've been really wonderful. You were wonderful today, and it was wonderful of you to come down here like this."

"Mom, I've got to say, now that I see you, I can't imagine how you thought you were going to manage without me or without somebody here."

"I don't know. I wasn't thinking, I guess."

"I just, I feel so bad." I don't know what it is I want to say, something about wishing I could do more. "I feel like I'm so unhappy myself that I'm more of a liability than anything else. Today, with Grandma, you know I nearly passed out at the dinner table?"

"Oh, Ellie, you were great today, you really were. Stop feeling bad about yourself. You've been wonderful to me."

"Mom, you know, it's just, it's so terrible, there's so much I'd like to do—" What am I trying to say? "There's just so much I'd like to do that I can't seem to do right now. I can't even finish a book lately. I'm barely in school, I'm not working, and I'm so drained it's as if I were working an eighty-hour week when in reality I'm tired from doing nothing. I can't even blame breaking up with Rafe for how bad I feel because I felt this way before I met him, and we weren't even together that long. I feel so lousy and there's nothing wrong with me and I have no excuse."

"But, Elizabeth," she says, in the most reasonable voice I've heard from her in years, "there is something wrong with you: You're depressed. That's a real problem. That's not imaginary. Of course you can't deal with anything. You're depressed."

I never knew that she understood. I'd never heard her acknowledge my depression so straightforwardly before. What had happened? Had somebody talked to her? Or was it all the painkillers she was taking? She almost never talked about anything that was wrong with me without qualifying it with a bunch of remarks about all the terrible things my father did to me and how he had ruined me and it was all his fault. She never could simply admit that I had a problem, it needed to be handled, who cares about pointing fingers and assigning blame. This was a definite first.

And it's strange, but when she said those words to me, when she said, *You're depressed*, it became a reality for me for the first time in a long, long time. Not that I wasn't aware that I felt like shit all the time—there was no avoiding that— but I had ceased to think of it as a legitimate condition, as a real disease, even if it did have a fancy diagnosis like *atypical depression*. No matter what Dr. Sterling or any of the other mental health practitioners ever said, I never felt I had a right to be depressed. I always felt like: Really, if I wanted to, I could snap out of this. And all the tenured faculty at Harvard Medical School could get together and tell me in their collective opinion that I had a real live chronic illness on my hands, and none of it would have meant as much as my mother telling me, for what I'm certain was the first time, that depression is a problem of its own that needs to be dealt with on its own terms.

I got up and sat next to her and hugged her, and thought to myself, She understands. She understands and it will be all right.

14

Think of Pretty Things

* * *

After they had explored all the suns in the universe,
and all the planets of all the suns, they realized that
there was no other life in the universe, and that they
were alone. And they were very happy, because then
they knew it was up to them to become all the things
they had imagined they would find.

LANFORD WILSON
Fifth of July

*On the plane back to school, I think that some insight is supposed
to be hitting me right now. Something about the meaning of life,
about dancing in the face of adversity, about struggling and persevering
and succeeding. Yes, I think, any minute now, before we touch down
into Logan, the insight will come. Clarity. The truth will set me free,
and all that.*

*Of course, it never happens. Years of therapy, and it never
happens. Psychotropic drugs, and it never happens. My mother gets
brutalized down the block from the building we live in, and it never
happens. That's the problem with reality, that's the fallacy of therapy: It assumes that you will have a series of revelations, or even just
one little one, and that these various truths will come to you and will
change your life completely. It assumes that insight alone is a transformative force. But the truth is, it doesn't work that way. In real
life, every day you might come to some new conclusion about yourself
and about the reasoning behind your behavior, and you can tell yourself that this knowledge will make all the difference. But in all like-*

lihood, you're going to keep on doing the same old things. You'll still be the same person. You'll still cling to your destructive, debilitating habits because your emotional tie to them is so strong—so much stronger than any dime-store insight you might come up with—that the stupid things you do are really the only things you've got that keep you centered and connected. They are the only things about you that make you you. For example, knowing you're attracted to men who are bad for you doesn't keep you from getting involved with men who are bad for you. It means only that you have new and improved ways to rationalize: *It's a father thing. Or, It's my way of reenacting my relationship with my mother's boyfriend who raped me when I was twelve. Or else, and this is the most desperate one, I'm like a drug addict, I need a fix, I can't help myself.*

If only life could be more like the movies, where characters muddle things through and do what's right in the end. But real life isn't like that. In Kramer vs. Kramer, *Meryl Streep thinks it over and decides to let her son stay with Dustin Hoffman, even though she's won their ugly custody battle; but in real life, what happens is more like the case of Baby M, where the grown-ups all fight it out in court and on national television, where no one thinks about what's right for the child, only about what they want and what the law allows, and in the end it's miserable. In* The Breakfast Club, *a geek, a jock, a rich bitch, a girl in black, and a hoodlum become best friends and reconcile their differences in a few hours' worth of detention; in real life, Saturday afternoon's momentary intimacy would result only in some forced, awkward exchanges on Monday morning, everyone returning to the same old cliques and clans, the same old lipstick shades and sunglasses.*

Yes, maybe years of therapy means that sooner or later, over time, you change your ways and yourself ever so slightly. But I don't have years. Or rather, it's already been years. I want it to be like the movies. I want an angel to swoop down to me like he does to

Jimmy Stewart in It's a Wonderful Life *and talk me out of suicide. Because at this point, that's what it's going to take.*

★   ★   ★

The suicide attempt startled even me. It seemed to happen out of context, like something that should have taken place months and months ago, when there was no hope at all, when Rafe and I first broke up, when England first turned into a rainy-day nightmare. It should never have happened within a few days of returning to Cambridge, at a point when, even I had to admit, the fluoxetine was starting to kick in. After all, I was able to get out of bed in the morning, which may not seem like much, but in my life it was up there with Moses parting the Red Sea. Suddenly, feeling like I ought to return the cash my mother gave me for London, I even found it within myself to walk up Brattle Street and over to a restaurant called the Harvest, where I was able to convince the manager that I had what it took to be a cashier and cappuccino maker. Anybody would have thought that these were signs that my mood was on the upswing, and I guess it was. But just as a little bit of knowledge is a dangerous thing, a little bit of energy, in the hands of someone hell-bent on suicide, is a very dangerous thing.

My improved affect did not in any way sway me from the philosophical conviction that life, at its height and at its depth, basically sucks. My mother's mugging really shook me up, and bad. It seemed impossible to reconcile with any concept of justice that something like this could happen to her, to someone whose whole life, in the first place, had never turned out quite the way she planned. Oh yes, I know, there are far more pitiful cases roaming the streets than my mother—homeless women, battered wives, hard-luck alcoholics who've lost their jobs, their families, their houses, their everything—but her particular tragedy was most striking to me, at least in part, because it really was so very banal. Here was a woman who should have had a house in the suburbs, a job she liked, involving either art or architecture, and a husband who cared for her, someone who owned a *shmata* company on Seventh Avenue or worked as a stockbroker or a middle manager at some large corporation like Procter & Gamble. That was all she wanted, nothing fancy, nothing like the kinds of stargazing dreams that I and everyone I know set their sights on. Instead, all she got was a daughter who is such a mental wreck that she is actually scared to answer the phone, never knowing what's going to happen next.

So the plan was simple: I would earn enough money to pay my mother back, and then I'd kill myself. I didn't care what drugs they put me on, I didn't care what state of false consciousness they were able to induce in me through chemicals. Because even if I wasn't depressed, I would still have years of more boyfriends who wouldn't work out to look forward to, I would still have a father who had no idea why I wouldn't talk to him, I would still have a whole world gone wrong to put up with, in which families disintegrate and relationships are meaningless. And I didn't want it.

I hate to admit it, but even after years of religious training I really don't believe in the afterlife. I still think that human beings, even our beautiful and wretched souls, are just biology, are just a series of chemical and physical reactions that one day stop, and so do we, and that is that. But I'm looking forward to this blank peace, this oblivion, this nothing, this not being me anymore. I am looking forward to it for real. Or at least, this is what I tell myself. I tell myself I'm not scared, I tell myself I really want to die, and it never occurs to me until the last possible moment that what I really want is to be saved.

It happens in Dr. Sterling's office. I see her on a Sunday (I have been seeing her just about every day because she is trying to keep me alive). I tell her that if I were to kill myself, I would get into a steaming hot bath in the dark, because in the dark you can't see what you are doing to yourself so you can't get scared and you can't scream, and I would slash my wrists and maybe a couple of other arteries with a fresh, shiny razor blade. And then I'd lie back in the tub and let it happen, let the blood and life drain out of me, to kingdom come and all that. I tell her that this is a surprisingly effective suicide method, from what I've read, and that the reason this kind of bloodletting so often fails is that people don't know that you've got to cut your wrists lengthwise, and not across, and because people keep the lights on, and get shocked by the sight of so much blood, and actually second-guess their decision. They also don't think of slitting their jugular vein, or some other major pulse point besides their wrists, to speed up the process. But I assure her that I won't make these mistakes.

I even imagine the perfect soundtrack for this event: not the obvious thing, strains of Janis Joplin and Billie Holiday wafting through the steamy air in the bathroom. That would be too much of a cliché, dying to the sounds of miserable women who wanted to die themselves, who *did* die themselves. Oh no, I'd be more original than that. I wouldn't even play my usual dolorous favorites, like the Velvet Underground or Joni Mitchell. Nor would I go for the demented-youth approach and put on some heavy metal, like those kids in Reno, Nevada, who blew their brains out with sawed-off shotguns while Judas Priest's *Stained Class* was playing. (When one of them survived—albeit with a bunch of silicone where his face used to be—he sued the band, claiming the lyrics made him do it.) I'd never do anything like that, and I would never taint my all-purpose favorites like Bob Dylan or Bruce Springsteen by playing them through my death, though one last listen to *Blood on the Tracks*, one last spin of *Darkness on the Edge of Town*, might be worth it before I actually began the cutting. Maybe better to stick to the Rolling Stones or the Beatles, a band I never liked, except for that one point in the beginning of "Strawberry Fields" when John Lennon sings, "Let me take you down . . ." Those are the words I want to leave the world with. *Let me take you down.* Down as low as I am. Yes, that's it, that's the plan, to die with John Lennon's voice seems just right.

As I discuss this scheme, I become downright rhapsodic, like a reformed coke addict going gaga over the thought of doing some blow, and Dr. Sterling looks at me like I'm giving her the creeps. "Look, Elizabeth, if you can detail these plans for me, I'm not letting you go home," she says. "I can't let you kill yourself. I'm going to take you to the hospital."

"I didn't say I would definitely do it."

"I know. But you're always complaining that no one takes your cries for help seriously. You've always said that you'd like to attempt suicide so that people would finally believe you need help." She sighs. "Well, I believe you. And you don't have to do something messy and dangerous to get the help you need. We can take you to the hospital now. I happen to know, because one of my other patients is suicidal, that there are no beds available in Westwood Lodge right now." She is referring to a hospital affiliated with McLean. "There might be room in Mt. Auburn, which is right nearby so I could work pretty closely with you. We can hop in the car and be there in two minutes."

Dr. Sterling matter-of-factly presents me with my options, and they all sound unbearable. She's not even mentioning Stillman anymore, she's talking about a real lock-up. And I can't have that. I feel panicky, scared of this confinement, even though I know perfectly well that whether I'm in a hospital or out roaming around, I am always so far from free because I am always enslaved to the caprices of my own mind or the whims of what the world has to offer. Even so,

I really don't want to be put away. I can't let her check me in, so I must check myself out. There is no logic to the suicide imperative, it is just something that I must do, and something I must do right now. I think of those lines in the Anne Sexton poem "Wanting to Die," in which she says that the urge to kill herself is with her always, even when she has nothing against life, because after a certain point, it's not about having a reason: "Suicides have a special language," she writes. "Like carpenters they want to know *which tools*. They never ask *why build*." So what tools do I have at my disposal? Nothing much, nothing terribly lethal, just a full bottle of Mellaril that I carry around in my knapsack at all times, just in case. In case what? Oh, I don't know, in case a moment like this occurs.

I ask Dr. Sterling if I can run to the bathroom, as if I were in preschool. She nods in assent and gathers her car keys. I grab my bag and run up the flight of stairs from her basement office and I feel suddenly liberated. I keep telling myself over and over again that I am going to be fine, and of course, I really am fine, as fine as I can be knowing that this is the end. I open the bathroom door, lock myself in, find the bottle of Mellaril and pour all the pills into my hand, open my mouth, and swallow them.

I have become pretty proficient at taking pills without water, without anything to wash them down, but I stand at the sink and cup my hands under the tap and swallow what I can, knowing the Mellaril will metabolize more easily with some liquid. There really aren't that many pills, a whole bunch, a handful big enough that a couple slip onto the floor, but I have to admit it's probably not a lethal dose, that I am probably doing exactly the thing I don't want to do, committing the act I believed I was above: making a wimpy attempt that is bound to fail. I don't know what kind of damage these will do me, maybe I'll sleep for a few days as I did at summer camp, maybe the pills will turn my head to blotto for a little while. My thoughts wander, almost soothingly, and I curl up, bend my knees, and pull my thighs to my chest, bunching myself up under the bathroom sink. I decide I will never leave this position or this place for as long as I have the choice.

But then I hear noises, Dr. Sterling banging on the bathroom door, pounding, pounding, pounding, saying, Come out, Elizabeth, come out! And finally I reach up my hand and unlock the door, and she finds me with the empty bottle beside me, and says, "Come on, we're going to the emergency room."

Once in the car, I start nodding off and feeling nauseous. I don't want to throw up but I have a feeling that's what I'm going to do. "I've never lost a patient before," Dr. Sterling says. "I'm not going to start now."

"Well, I hope you're not doing this for the sake of your statistics." And then I realize what a horrible thing that is to say to her. She has visited me in the infirmary, she's taken my phone calls at 3:00 A.M., and now she's driving me to the emergency room, and the only reason she's done any of this is that she cares. The Mellaril is definitely kicking in big time, but I don't want to be rude, I don't want the last thing I say to her before slipping into some kind of coma to be something snide. "I'm sorry. That was a terrible thing to say." And then my head falls against the window in a deep daze.

As soon as I walk through the automatic glass doors in the entrance to the emergency room, falling on Dr. Sterling's shoulder, barely able to stand straight, I feel myself choking. Some small remnant of vanity takes over, and I make my way into the bathroom, fall into a stall, and vomit, watch a mess of orange drip out of my mouth. Lots of pills, some of them have maintained the integrity of their round, tablet shape, but most of them are spewing, melting, disintegrating, falling apart, a surrealistic vision in shades of tan and salmon as they flush down the toilet. All I can think to say when I walk out and see Dr. Sterling talking to one of the doctors is, "I guess I won't be getting my stomach pumped. This experience just won't be complete." I start to laugh and laugh as if this were the funniest thing I've ever said. I feel absolutely euphoric—wasted and spent, but still euphoric. *I have survived an attempt on my life.* What a strange, nervous thing that is. So I laugh some more as the doctor leads me into one of the examining rooms, orange spittle beginning to cake on my chin.

Dr. Sterling gets on the phone with the head psychiatrist at Harvard and starts explaining my condition, explaining that she knows there are no beds at Westwood Lodge because another one of her other charges wanted to go there. I have no idea what he said in response, but suddenly she laughs. "Well, you know how it is, me and all my suicidal patients."

I am stunned to hear Dr. Sterling speaking of me as if she were a grocer discussing a shipment of rotten apples. Shoptalk, I guess. But Jesus. *Hah hah hah, me and all my suicidal patients are partying at Westwood Lodge.* I guess even psychiatrists are entitled to gallows humor.

In the course of the phone conversation, the two doctors determine that it's all right for me to stay at Stillman for the night, but after that they have to send me to a real hospital. The infirmary is not equipped to deal with suicidal patients. In the meantime, the doctor at Stillman will have to arrange for a police officer to guard my room and make sure I don't try to kill myself. Suicide is, apparently, an illegal act.

"A *policeman*?!" I gasp at Dr. Sterling as she explains this to me. By this time I am lying on a table in a small room, a place that looks familiar. Is this where they took me when I miscarried? "What am I? A criminal? I'm not armed and dangerous or anything. I'm just unhappy."

"I know that," she says. "And I trust that if you tell me you won't hurt yourself, you won't. I believe in nonsuicide pacts. But if you're going to stay here, they have to do what they think is necessary to protect you and protect themselves."

"I see." For a moment I am amused that with all the crime and assorted disaster there is in Cambridge, the police department is going to waste an officer on me, but I try not to think about it. I feel pretty good suddenly, as if I am having some kind of postoverdose rush. Of course, I also feel pretty bad. I feel all over the map, strange and wandering in some emotional diaspora that no previous experience has ever prepared me for. To deliberately hurt yourself is too counterintuitive. It's not as if I've never been self-destructive before, but it was always in the context of trying to make life more bearable, to make living through some sad moment more tolerable. But a deliberate overdose is not part of a night out or a party: It is self-destruction for its own sake, and it is consequently the purest and most deliberate act of hatred I have ever committed. It doesn't matter if I never really figured on dying: I still feel that I've crossed a line, and that in doing so I now can actually return from the other side of that border. A sudden and nearly manic lust for life overcomes me. I lie there and feel this strange urge to go home and jump on my bed, to yell at no one in particular that hah hah hah I'm still alive.

While I'm lying in bed at Stillman watching *60 Minutes*, Dr. Sterling calls to check on me. I tell her that I want this to be the last night I ever spend in Stillman, that the place has become positively hateful to me, that it reeks of a person I don't want to be. I am so tired of the girl in the infirmary, I am so sick of the girl who cries wolf all the time—even though not one of those cries was ever a false alarm. Not one of my pleas for help was ever less than truly urgent because when it's all in your mind, there always *is* a wolf. That's what it feels like,

I try to explain: This wolf has been stalking me for ten years, and now it's time he went away. Time for me to get better.

"So you believe in the possibility now?" she asks.

"Well, yes. Maybe." No. "A definite maybe. It's just that I took this fairly serious suicidal action today, and I guess I realize that I don't want to die. I don't want to live either, but—" There really isn't anything in-between. Depression is about as close as you get to somewhere between dead and alive, and it's the worst. "But since the tendency toward inertia means that it's easier for me to stay alive than die, I guess that's how it's going to be, so I guess I should try to be happy."

"That sounds right."

"Look, I don't have a lot of faith in this life business." Always making disclaimers. "But, you know, I think I'm stuck."

"Listen, Elizabeth," Dr. Sterling says. "I just spoke to your mother."

"You didn't!"

"I didn't tell her about what happened, but I told her you were particularly down right now and having a very hard time. And she asked me what she should do." Pregnant pause. "She doesn't know what to do. She'd really like to help you, but she's afraid. She doesn't really understand, but I know she's trying."

"Oh."

"Maybe you should call her. She was going to try to reach you at Stillman, but maybe you should get in touch with her first. I don't really know what to say about her." Very pregnant pause. "I know that she really loves you and she wants you to be all right. It's just hard for her. Hard for everybody."

"Yeah," I say. "I know. Look, you're not under any legal obligation to report this to her, are you?"

"No."

"Well, good. Don't." I can't imagine what my mother would do if she'd heard I'd taken an overdose. She might take one too. She might kill me. "Listen, Dr. Sterling?"

"Uh-huh?"

"You're not going to lock me away, are you? Because I don't want that."

"I've never wanted that for you, Elizabeth." She sighs. "I always believed you could get better some other way. I still think the fluoxetine will work soon."

"It's working already."

"Well, then why did you do what you did earlier?"

It's such a hard question. It seems like such a trifling, frivolous act to have committed only so that I could lie here watching *60 Minutes* an hour later. "I think I wanted to know," I try. "I wanted to know what it felt like to go that far. I wanted to brush with death to see if I'd like it better. But you know, there was a moment when I was sitting in your car, and the Mellaril was hitting, and I thought to myself that maybe this will work after all, maybe I really will die, and I didn't like that idea at all. I started thinking about all these things I had to do. You know, I thought to myself that I'm supposed to go back to Dallas this summer, I'm supposed to hand in my junior essay, I'm supposed to have this future ahead of me that's so—" I had to stop myself because I was about to say *full of promise*, those unbearable words, those lying, cheating words that no one can ever live up to. But of course, they described exactly what was supposed to happen, what was supposed to be happening all along.

"And this may sound kind of stupid, but I kept thinking," I continue, "that they can't lock me away because soon it will be summer and I don't think they have Steve's ice cream at McLean. You know, I started to think about all these little things, and I thought, damn it, I can't die yet. They weren't terribly grand thoughts, just mundane pleasures that I still had to look forward to. I guess this sounds so dumb." Dr. Sterling starts to say something about how any reason one finds to stay alive is as worthy as any other, but I'm still embarrassed to be talking about ice cream now.

"I wish I could say something more profound, but I don't know if there really is anything so grand in my future," I try. "But I know for a fact that no matter what else goes wrong, there are still a few things I will always like doing, you know, like listening to Springsteen or seeing the movie *Nashville* yet again or going to Greta Garbo double features or putting on Glenn Gould's 1955 recording of the *Goldberg Variations* or buying a new lipstick. It's all such simple stuff, but it matters. You know, the worst thing about depression is that not even the small pleasures can offer any tiny bit of comfort. At best, they're kind of okay. I mean, if Noah and I *had* found clams in Ipswich, I'm sure it wouldn't have made me happy at all. It would have been one more failed attempt. But now, you know, I feel so relieved to be alive that I want to take in a few little indulgences. I feel like I should go get a Heath Bar Crunch cone."

"That's actually not an atypical response to a suicide attempt," Dr. Sterling says. "The aftermaths vary so much. Some people really do deteriorate and get worse because their attempts occur much earlier on in their treatment. Some people only *begin* treatment after they've taken an overdose and are forced to. But in your case, it seems to have been something you did as a last attempt to hold on to the person you have been for so many years, the person who's depressed all the time. You're the one who's always saying that without depression, you'd have no personality at all. Well, I really think that the fluoxetine is going to work, and that whole part of you is going to go away. And I think you're scared. I think you're trying to tell me that even if you get better, it doesn't mean that you don't need me anymore, and it doesn't mean you don't need therapy and help and care anymore. Typically, in your household, the only way anything got attended to was if it had reached a point of complete desperation. But, Elizabeth, trust me, you don't need to be desperate in order for me to help you. I'm still going to be here for you even if you're not suicidally depressed."

And, for what seems like the eighth time that day, I start to cry.

In a strange way, I had fallen in love with my depression. Dr. Sterling was right about that. I loved it because I thought it was all I had. I thought depression was the part of my character that made me worthwhile. I thought so little of myself, felt that I had such scant offerings to give to the world, that the one thing that justified my existence at all was my agony. Taking a hypersensitive approach to life had come to seem so much more pure and honest than joining the ranks of the numb masses who could let it all slide by. What I'd stopped realizing was that if you feel everything intensely, ultimately you feel nothing at all. Everything registers at the same decibel so that the death of a roach crawling across a Formica counter can seem as tragic as the death of your own father. The people on the outside— and that's the right word, because to a depressive everyone else is outside—who are selectively expending their emotional energy are actually a lot more honest than anyone who is depressed and has replaced all nuance with a constant, persistent, droning despair.

But depression gave me more than just a brooding introspection. It gave me humor, it gave me a certain what-a-fuck-up-I-am schtick to play with when the worst was over. I couldn't kid myself and think that anyone enjoyed my tears and hysteria—plainly, they didn't—but the side effects, the by-products of depression, seemed to keep me going. I had developed a persona that could be extremely melodramatic and entertaining. It had, at times, all the selling points of madness, all the aspects of performance art. I was always able to reduce whatever craziness I'd experienced into the perfect anecdote, the ideal cocktail party monologue, and until that final year of real lows, I think most people would have said that when I wasn't being carted off to the emergency room I was fun. Even at my worst, when people came to see me at Stillman, I would try to keep the atmosphere light by saying something like, So, did I tell you about the accidental blowjob?

Anyway, I thought this ability, to tell away my personal life as if it didn't belong to me, to be queerly chatty and energetic at moments that most people found inappropriate, was what my friends liked about me. In fact, over time, in the years of my recovery from depression, most of them let me know, one by one, that while they didn't mind *that I said things that were thoughtless and out of line, they excused this behavior as a sad flaw. It wasn't what they liked about me at all. It was what they put up with, because when I wasn't busy flying around the room and ranting about nothing, I was actually just good to talk to, even a good friend. That's all their feelings for me were about. They'd be just as happy to see all the affectation go.*

But before I knew this, I was so scared to give up depression, fearing that somehow the worst part of me was actually all of me. The idea of throwing away my depression, of having to create a whole personality, a whole way of living and being that did not contain misery as its leitmotif, was daunting. Depression had for so long been a convenient—and honest—explanation for everything that was wrong with me, and it had been a handicap that helped accentuate everything that was right. Now, with the help of a biochemical cure, it was going to go away. I mean, wild animals raised in captivity will perish if placed back into their natural habitats because they don't know the laws of prey and predator and they don't know the ways of the jungle, even if that's where they belong. How would I ever survive as my normal *self? And after all these years, who was that person anyway?*

The day after the suicide attempt, Dr. Sterling lets me leave Stillman, and I get up and go to work at the Harvest as if nothing is wrong. It is my first day, and it is pretty clear as the manager tries to show me how to tilt a decanter of milk in different ways to produce different consistencies of steam, that this is one in a series of menial jobs I will miserably fail at. Nonetheless, I am almost happy to be behind the cash register and in front of the coffee maker today. I'm happy to be doing anything routine and normal.

At some point, when things slow down during lunch, I call Dr. Sterling to tell her I feel strange and lonely because my friends were mostly angry at me about what had happened. Eben insisted that he felt just as bad as me sometimes and didn't do things like that. Alec lectured me about how I had let myself fall into this funk and he wasn't surprised that I felt so awful considering I'd wrecked my life by spending most of first semester in Rhode Island and most of second semester in California and England. Everybody I'd spoken to about the overdose in its immediate aftermath was almost mean about it. I had expected some version of sympathy, and instead people kept telling me I'd brought this on myself. From the way they were talking, you'd think I'd committed murder—not attempted suicide. Even Samantha, my bedrock, my sob sister, seemed annoyed. I think she said, What a stupid thing to do!

Dr. Sterling explains that this is normal. She says people can be understanding about almost anything but suicide. "Remember," she says, "these are people who feel like they're doing the best they can to be helpful, and you do something that indicates your utter rejection and dissatisfacton with their efforts. It's infuriating."

After I hang up the receiver, I return to one waiter demanding a double espresso, a decaf cappuccino, and a café au lait, while another wants two espressos, a decaf double espresso, and a tea, and everyone needs to deliver the orders at once, everyone is shouting at me at once, I can't remember what anyone says, and I think: What if they knew? Just as I walked around the day after I lost my virginity, wondering if my aspect had changed, if my cheeks revealed this new experience in a rosier glow, today I wonder if people know I'm a failed suicide.

And then something just kind of changed in me. Over the next few days, I became all right, safe in my own skin. It happened just like that. One morning I woke up, and I really did want to live, really looked forward to greeting the day, imagined errands to run, phone calls to return, and it was not with a feeling of great dread, not with the sense that the first person who stepped on my toe as I walked through the square may well have driven me to suicide. It was as if the miasma of depression had lifted off me, gone smoothly about its business, in the same way that the fog in San Francisco rises as the day wears on. Was it the Prozac? No doubt. Was it the cathartic nature of going through a suicide attempt? Probably. Just as I always said that I went down gradually and then suddenly, I also got up that way. All the therapy, all the traveling, all the sleeping, all the drugs, all the crying, all the missed classes, all the lost time—all of that was part of some slow recovery process that came to the end of its tether at the same time that I reached mine.

It took a long time for me to get used to my contentedness. It was so hard for me to formulate a way of being and thinking in which the starting point was not depression. Dr. Sterling agrees that it's hard, because depression is an addiction the way many substances and most modes of behavior are, and like most addictions it is miserable but still hard to break. On Prozac, I often walk around so conscious of how not-terrible I feel that I am petrified that I'm going to lose this new equilibrium. I spend so much time worrying about staying happy that I threaten to become unhappy all over again. Any time I am bothered about anything, whether it's a line that's too long at the bank or a man who doesn't return my love, I have to remind myself that these emotional experiences (petty annoyance in the former instance, heartbreak in the latter) are reasonable and discrete unto themselves. They don't have to precipitate a depressive episode. It takes me a long time to realize that when I get upset about something it doesn't mean that the tears will never stop. It is so hard to learn to put sadness in perspective, so hard to understand that it is a feeling that comes in degrees, it can be a candle burning gently and harmlessly in your home, or it can be a full-fledged forest fire that destroys almost everything and is controlled by almost nothing. It can also be so much in-between.

In-between. There's a phrase that is far too underappreciated. What a great day it was, what a moment of pure triumph, to have discovered that there are in-betweens. What freedom it is to live in a spectral world that most people take for granted. Being somewhere in the middle is anathema in our culture, it connotes mediocrity, middlingness, an item that is so-so, okay, not bad, not good, not much of anything. So many people feel a need to go bungee jumping or to take vacations in Third World countries full of scorpions and armed dictators. So many people spend so much time in adventures meant only to take them out of that boring middle range, that placid emotional state where it feels, no doubt, like nothing ever happens. But me, all I want is that nice even keel. All I want is a life where the extremes are in check, where I am in check.

All I want is to live in between.

I will never not be on guard for depression, but the constancy, the obsessive and totalizing effect of that disease, the sense that life is something happening to other people I am watching through an opaque cloud, is gone.

The black wave, for the most part, is gone.

On a good day, I don't even think about it anymore.

It's funny, but when I was little, before I'd go to sleep my mom would do this routine with me where she'd tell me to think of pretty things. I would close my eyes and she would run her fingers over my cheeks and across my brow. And we'd go through this list. I think it was a way of preventing nightmares—and it would always be, you know, pussycats and puppy dogs and balloons at the zoo. Sometimes she'd mention yellow submarines, stars in the sky, blackbirds flying overhead, trees in Central Park, and even—believe it or not—that on Saturday I would get to see Daddy. Nothing that extraordinary, but when you're four years old, it's cats and dogs that make life worth living. And I kind of think it's maybe not so different now.

Epilogue: Prozac Nation
✳ ✳ ✳

Not too long ago, my friend Olivia brought her cat to the veterinarian because she was chewing clumps of fur off her back and vomiting all the time. The doctor looked at Isabella and immediately diagnosed the animal with something called excessive grooming disorder, which meant that the cat had grown depressed and self-absorbed, perhaps because Olivia's boyfriend had moved out of the apartment, perhaps because Olivia was traveling so much. At any rate, the vet explained, this was an obsessive-compulsive disorder. Isabella couldn't stop cleaning herself just as certain people can't stop vacuuming their apartments, or washing their hands all the time like Lady Macbeth. The vet recommended treating the cat with Prozac, which had proved extremely effective in curing this condition in humans. A feline-size prescription was administered.

Now, you have to understand that Olivia had been on and off Prozac and its chemical variants for a couple of years herself, hoping to find a way to cope with her constant bouts of depression. Olivia had also recently insisted that her boyfriend either go on Prozac or take a hike because his sluggishness and foul moods were destroying their relationship. And I had, of course, been on Prozac for more than six years at that point. So when she called to tell me that now Isabella was on it too, we laughed. "Maybe that's what my cat needs," I joked. "I mean, he's been under the weather lately."

There was a nervous edge to our giggling.

"I think this Prozac thing has gone too far," Olivia said.

"Yes." I sighed. "Yes, I think it has."

I never thought that depression could seem funny, never thought there'd be a time when I could be amused thinking that of the $1.3 billion spent on prescriptions for Prozac last year (up about thirty percent since 1992), some of them might even be for our household pets, who are apparently as susceptible to mental trauma as the rest of us. I never thought I would amazedly read about Wenatchee, Washington, a town known as "The Apple Capital of the World," a place where six hundred out of its twenty-one thousand residents are all on Prozac, and where one psychologist has come to be known as "The Pied Piper of Prozac." I never thought that the *New York Times*, reporting on the eleven million people who have taken Prozac—six million in the United States alone—would declare on its front page that this consitituted a "legal drug culture." I never thought there would be so many cartoons with Prozac themes in *The New Yorker*, illustrating, among other things, a serotonin-happy Karl Marx declaring, "Sure! Capitalism can work out its kinks!" I never thought that in the same week I would stare down at both a *Newsweek* cover with a large, missile-like capsule beneath the caption "Beyond Prozac" and a *New Republic* cover of some shiny, happy peo-

ple enjoying their sunny lives above the headline "That Prozac Moment!"

I never thought that this antidote to a disease as serious
as depression—a malady that easily could have ended my
life—would become a national joke.

Since I first began taking Prozac, the pill has become the
second most commonly prescribed drug in this country (behind Zantac, the ulcer remedy), with one million orders filled
by pharmacists each month. Back in 1990, the story of this
wonder drug made the covers of many national periodicals.
Rolling Stone deemed Prozac the "hot yuppie upper," and all
the major network newsmagazines and daytime talk shows
began to do their Prozac-saved-my-life segments. In 1993,
when *Listening to Prozac*, Peter Kramer's book of case studies
and meditations on Prozac as a pill that could transform personality, entered the *New York Times* bestseller list for a six-
month stay, a new crop of cover stories and television pieces
appeared all over again. Dr. Kramer even referred to the pub-
licity jaunt for his book as the "Three Degrees of Separation
Tour" because it seemed that no one was more than three
people removed from someone on Prozac. While a backlash
of reports, mostly promulgated by the Church of Scientology,
linked Prozac with incidents of suicide and murder, the many
people that it relieved from symptoms of depression had nothing but praise. Cheryl Wheeler, a New England folkie, even
wrote a song called "Is It Peace or Is It Prozac?"

But all this coverage is not just about Prozac. It's about
the mainstreaming of mental illness in general and depression
in particular. It is about the way a state of mind once considered tragic has become completely commonplace, even worthy of comedy. It seemed that suddenly, some time in 1990,
I ceased to be this freakishly depressed person who had scared
the hell out of people for most of my life with my mood
swings and tantrums and crying spells, and I instead became

downright trendy. This private world of loony bins and weird people that I had always felt I occupied and hid in had suddenly been turned inside out so that it seemed like this was one big Prozac Nation, one big mess of malaise. In a quote in *Good Housekeeping* (good God, a magazine your grandmother reads), the psychologist Ellen McGrath described dysthymia as "the common cold of mental experience," noting that this form of chronic low-grade despair afflicts three percent of Americans (roughly the same number of people who have taken Prozac). I realize that to say that we live in the United States of Depression would surely indicate a skewed perception—the twelve million people said to be suffering from the illness is still a minority—but talk of depression as the mental disease of our times has been very much in the air these last few years, and has almost become a political issue. When Hillary Rodham Clinton campaigned on behalf of what a cover story in *New York Times Magazine* deemed "The Politics of Virtue," it was hard not to notice that her references to a "sleeping sickness of the soul," to "alienation and despair and hopelessness," to a "crisis of meaning," and to a "spiritual vacuum" seemed to imply that the country's problems have less to do with taxes and unemployment than with the simple fact that we were in one big collective bad mood. It almost seemed as if, perhaps, the next time half a million people gather for a protest march on the White House green it will not be for abortion rights or gay liberation, but because we're all so bummed out.

Of course, one of the striking elements of this depression breakout is the extent to which it has gotten such a strong hold on so many young people. The Miltown and Valium addicts of the fifties and sixties, the housewives reaching for their mother's little helpers, the strung out junkies and crackheads who litter the gutters of the Bowery or the streets of Harlem or the skid row of any town—all of these people were stereotyped as wasted, dissipated, and middle-aged, or else young and going nowhere fast. What is fascinating about depression this time—what is unique about this Prozac Nation—is the extent to which it is affecting those who have so much to look forward to and to hope for, who are, as one might say of any bright young thing about to make her debut into the world, so full of promise. These are people about whom one cannot say that life is over, that it's already too late, but rather young people for whom it has just begun.

On December 8, 1992, an article appeared in the science section of the *New York Times* under the headline "A Rising Cost of Modernity: Depression." The piece tells of a report published by the *Journal of the American Medical Association*, which delivered the results of a long-term, international, multigenerational study of depression. The main point: Those born after 1955 are *three times* as likely as their grandparents' generation to suffer from depression. In fact, of Americans born before 1905, only one percent had experienced a depressive episode by age seventy-five, while of those born after 1955, six percent were already depressed by age twenty-four. Apparently, the trend is global, with studies in Italy, Germany, Taiwan, Lebanon, Canada, France, New Zealand, Puerto Rico, and elsewhere yielding similar numbers. While women are thought to be two or three times as likely as men to get depressed, the article concludes that "the gap between men and women in rates of depression is narrowing among younger generations, with the risk in young men beginning to rise to the levels seen in women." In the end, the article concedes that the increased incidence of depression could be partly explained by a greater openness about the topic, but these statistics are so alarming that experts think candor is not much of a factor.

In the meantime, the anecdotal evidence would seem to bear out the point that a lot of people are either truly depressed, or they believe themselves to be. And many think that Prozac is the answer. We've all heard stories like the one about the burglar who left the computer, VCR, and stereo equipment untouched, but ran off with the bottle of Prozac. Or perhaps, like me, you've been in the unfortunate position of being in the back seat of a taxi while the driver confesses that a few months ago he tried to kill himself with a hundred Valium pills and a whiskey chaser, but now he's on Prozac and life couldn't be better. Maybe you find out that the guy who fixes your plumbing is on Prozac, that your gynecologist is on Prozac, that your boss is on Prozac, that your mother is on Prozac, maybe your grandmother too. Even if Prozac has not seeped into your personal life in some way, many of the famous and infamous have confessed to being users. Gary Hart was on Prozac for a while. Jim Bakker has tried it. Roseanne Arnold is on it. Jeffrey Dahmer just took himself off it.

How is it possible that so many are so miserable?

I know there are people who get a kick out of this kind of thing. They enter twelve-step fellowships so that they can find others afflicted with the same demons: alcoholism, narcotics addiction, eating disorders, and a plethora of imaginary illnesses like shopping, loving, or fucking too much. But it seems to me that there's something wrong with a world where all these pills are circulating, floating around the atmosphere like a spreading virus or bad information or mean gossip. I have no way to be certain of this, but my guess is that most of the people on Prozac haven't taken the circuitous path to this drug that I did. Many general practitioners give Prozac to patients without much thought. In a 1993 study, researchers at the Rand Corporation found that more than half of the physicians they surveyed got out their prescription pads after discussing depression with a patient for *less* than three minutes. Sometimes I find myself resenting the ease with which doctors now perform this bit of pharmacologic prestidigitation. By the time I was put on Prozac they'd tried everything else possible, I'd had my brain fried and blunted with so many other drugs, I'd spent over a decade in a prolonged state of clinical despair. Nowadays, Prozac seems to be a panacea available for the asking.

Still, I can't ignore the compelling evidence presented in the *New York Times* article that would seem to indicate that maybe all this drug prescribing is not an overaggressive response, but actually a sane reaction on the part of doctors to a whole slew of people for whom simple existence is fraught with intense misery. According to a study done by the *Journal of Clinical Psychiatry*, in 1990 alone 290 million work days were lost to depression. The same report also states that depression costs this country $43.7 billion annually, a figure that includes the price of psychiatric care as well as losses incurred by impaired productivity and worker absence. If we added in the amount of money wasted by doctors requesting unnecessary lab tests because they've mistaken depression for some other disease, or if we tacked on the cost of adjunct treatments—drug abuse rehabilitation, for instance—the number would be much higher. Furthermore, on National Depression Awareness Day, when screening sites are set up all over the country to examine people for symptoms of major depression, fifty percent of those tested (admittedly a self-selected bunch) are found to be clinical cases. With all these statistics flying around, subjective though they may be, who's to say that there's too much Prozac? Maybe there isn't enough. Maybe this world is too difficult to negotiate without some kind of chemical buffer zone.

And while depression is a problem for any age group, the sense of it as a normal state of mind, as an average part of getting through the day, as so much ho-hum life-sucks-and-then-you-die, does seem unique to people who are now in their twenties and thirties. There is a certain shading to the dead-end depression of youth culture, some quality of fatalism about it, a resignation that makes it frighteningly banal. It is no wonder that something as similarly uninspired as Prozac, a pill that doesn't make you happy but does make you not sad, would become the drug of choice for this condition. No other substance feels quite so safe.

When I was reading a copy of *Lear's* in the Miami Beach sun, I chanced upon an article titled "The Plot Sickens," in which Fanny Howe, a college writing instructor, says that the gruesome, pessimistic nature of her students' submissions is like nothing she's seen in twenty-one years of teaching. "To read their work, you'd think they were a generation that was starved, beaten, raped, arrested, addicted, and war-torn. Inexplicable intrusions of random tragedy break up the otherwise good life of the characters," Howe writes. "The figures in their fictions are victims of hideous violence by accident; they commit crimes, but only for the hell of it; they hate, not understanding why they hate; they are loved or abused or depressed, and don't know why. . . . Randomness rules."

And Howe seems surprised by what she's reading. For me, and for everyone I know my age, such stories seem normal, peculiarly ordinary. In the world that we live in, randomness does rule. And this lack of order is a debilitating, destabilizing thing. Perhaps what has come to be placed in the catchall category of depression is really a guardedness, a nervousness, a suspicion about intimacy, any of many perfectly natural reactions to a world that seems to be perilously lacking in the basic guarantees that our parents expected: a marriage that would last, employment that was secure, sex that wasn't deadly. It is a cliché at this point to make reference to the economic and social insecurity that is said to characterize a mass of people that's been known collectively as Generation X or twentynothings, but obviously there is a lot of unhappiness going around in this age group, and I can't blame journalists, sociologists, and other observers for trying to make sense of it, for rooting out the causes.

The trouble is that when we get around to solutions, always seems to come down to Prozac. Or Zoloft or Pax Deep clinical depression is a disease, one that not only ca but probably should, be treated with drugs. But a low-grad terminal anomie, a sense of alienation or disgust and detach ment, the collective horror at a world that seems to have gon so very wrong, is not a job for antidepressants. The trouble is, the big-picture problems that have so many people down are more or less insoluble: As long as people *can* get divorced they *will* get divorced; America's shrinking economy is not reversible; there is no cure for AIDS. So it starts to seem fairly reasonable to anesthetize ourselves in the best possible way. I would like so much to say that Prozac is preventing many people who are not clinically depressed from finding real antidotes to what Hillary Clinton refers to as "a sleeping sickness of the soul," but what exactly would those solutions be? I mean, universal health care coverage and a national service draft would be nice, but neither one is going to save us from ourselves. Just as our parents quieted us when we were noisy by putting us in front of the television set, maybe we're now learning to quiet our own adult noise with Prozac.

And yet, I can't escape the icky feeling I get every time I'm sitting in a full car and everyone but the driver is on Prozac. I can't get away from some sense that after years of trying to get people to take depression seriously—of saying, I have a *disease*, I *need* help—now it has gone beyond the point of recognition as a real problem to become something that appears totally trivial. One of the creepiest moments for me was discovering that six million Americans had taken Prozac. As a Jew, I had always associated that precise number with something else entirely. How would I come to reinterpret *six mil-*

lion, to associate it with something quite different, a statistic that ought to be frightening but instead starts to seem rather ridiculous?

Every so often, I find myself with the urge to make sure people know that I am not just on Prozac but on lithium too, that I am a real sicko, a depressive of a much higher order than all these happy-pill poppers with their low-level sorrow. Or else I feel compelled to remind people that I've been on Prozac since the F.D.A. first approved it, that I've been taking it longer than anyone else on earth, save for a few laboratory rats in cages, trapped but happy. I don't know if I ought to be more dismayed by my need for Prozac one-upmanship, or by the fact that it isn't entirely unwarranted. After all, the media phenomenon of Prozac is such that it's turning a serious problem into a joke at a point when that really should not be happening: By most accounts, two-thirds of the people with severe depression are not being treated for it. And they are the ones who are likely to get lost in the rhetoric.

As Prozac becomes viewed as a silly drug for crybabies, an instrument of what Dr. Kramer calls "cosmetic pharmacology," the people whom it might really help—the ones who *need* it—will start to think that Prozac won't help them. In the rape-crisis debate that currently rages, many feminists argue that too loose a definition of rape results in not taking "real" rape seriously, while others claim that anyone who feels violated *was* violated—and what tends to get lost in all the screaming and yelling is that there are all these real people who are raped and are in terrible pain. It seems entirely possible to me now, given the tone of so many of the articles about Prozac, that people will forget how severe, crippling, and awful depression really is.

And I'm not the only one who's concerned. Eli Lilly and Company, the manufacturer that has profited bountifully from the excesses of Prozac, recently launched an advertising campaign in medical trade journals that begins with the head-line "Trivializing a Serious Illness." The ad first appeared in *Psychiatric News*, with copy that derides Prozac's "unprece-dented media attention in recent weeks," and declares that "much of this attention has trivialized the very serious nature of the disease Prozac was specifically developed to treat—clinical depression." In an article in the *Wall Street Journal*, Steven Paul, M.D., the head of central nervous system re-search at Eli Lilly, explains that the point of this ad is simply to help Prozac reach those who need it most. "Anything that confuses the appropriate use of Prozac or any of the antide-pressants in the mind of the public might scare people away from using the medication, or perhaps even scare physicians from prescribing it," Dr. Paul is quoted as saying. He adds that all the debate about whether Prozac can be used for subtle personality changes has "bogged down" efforts to get the drug out to the truly, deeply depressed.

While many of the people commenting in the *Journal* article suggested that the advertisement was the result of Eli Lilly's fear of liability suits as Prozac is overprescribed, or even because the corporation is concerned that the drug will be excluded from a national health care plan because it is seen as too frivolous, I'd like to believe that its aim might be honest. At two or three dollars a pill, at the rate of two pills a day, over a span of six years, I feel that I have already mortgaged my life to Eli Lilly. For the $11,000 worth of business I've given the company, I wouldn't mind believing that they're doing a little bit of public service.

The secret I sometimes think that only I know is that Prozac really isn't that great. Of course, I can say this and still believe that Prozac was the miracle that saved my life and jump-started me out of a full-time state of depression—which would probably seem to most people reason enough to think of the drug as manna from heaven. But after six years on Prozac, I know that it is not the end but the beginning. Mental health is so much more complicated than any pill that any mortal could invent. A drug, whether it's Prozac, Thorazine, an old-fashioned remedy like laudanum, or a street narcotic like heroin, can work only as well as the brain allows it to. And after a while, a strong, hardy, deep-seated depression will outsmart any chemical. While Prozac kept me pretty well leveled for the first several months I was on it, shortly thereafter I had a fight with my boyfriend in Dallas over Christmas. I took an overdose of Desyrel, an antidepressant I'd been given to supplement the Prozac, and ended up back in the emergency-room milieu that had once been so familiar to me. I hadn't poisoned myself terribly seriously (I'd taken about ten pills), and the hospital released me into the care of my boyfriend's parents. When I got back to Cambridge, Dr. Sterling put me on lithium, both to augment the effects of Prozac and to even out some extreme mood swings. Regardless of my diagnosis of atypical depression, she was starting to think I was maybe cyclothymic or manic-depressive after all, going from gleeful revelry one day to suicidal gestures the next.

I stopped taking Desyrel once I started on lithium, but all my attempts to lower my Prozac dose have resulted in an onset of the same old symptoms. I have occasionally tried to go off of lithium altogether, because it is a draining, tiring drug to take, but those attempts to cut it out inevitably lead to scenes like the one that found me spilled across my bathroom and wrecked out in tears and black chiffon after we'd had that huge party at our house. At times, even on both lithium and Prozac, I have had severe depressive episodes, ones that kept my friends in a petrified all-night vigil while I refused to get up off the kitchen floor, refused to stop crying, refused to relinquish the grapefruit knife I gripped in my hand

and pointed at my wrist. After these difficult scenes, when I finally come to enough to seek medical help, the psycho-pharmacologist invariably will decide to put me on some additional drug like desipramine, or he will suggest I try taking Desyrel once again, or he will even ask if occasional use of Mellaril might not be what I really need.

Just as many germs have outsmarted antibiotics such that diseases like tuberculosis, once thought to be under control, have reemerged in newer, more virulent mutant strains, so depression manages to reconfigure itself so that it is more than just a matter of too little serotonin. As Susanna Kaysen points out in *Girl, Interrupted*, her memoir of a stay at McLean Hospital, "It's a long way from not having enough serotonin to thinking that the world is 'stale, flat and unprofitable'; even further to writing a play about a man driven by that thought. That leaves a lot of mind room. Something is interpreting the clatter of neurological activity." Of course, those interpretations may well be the result of still more neurological activity, but it might be the kind that is not amenable to outside scientific intervention. I believe, perhaps superstitiously, although my experience completely confirms it, that brain cells will always outsmart medical molecules. If you are chronically down, it is a lifelong fight to keep from sinking.

In the case of my own depression, I have gone from a thorough certainty that its origins are in bad biology to a more flexible belief that after an accumulation of life events made my head such an ugly thing to be stuck in, my brain's chemicals started to agree. There's no way to know any of this for sure right now. There isn't some blood test, akin to those for mononucleosis or HIV, that you can take to find a mental imbalance. And the anecdotal evidence leads only to a lot of chicken-and-egg types of questions: After all, depression does run in my family, but that might just be because we're all subject to being raised by other depressives. Where my depression is concerned, the fact that Prozac in combination with other drugs has been, for the most part, a successful antidote, leads me to believe that regardless of how I got started on my path of misery, by the time I got treatment the problem was certainly chemical. What many people don't realize is that the cause-and-effect relationship in mental disorders is a two-way shuttle: It's not just that an a priori imbalance can make you depressed. It's that years and years of exogenous depression (a malaise caused by external events) can actually fuck up your internal chemistry so much that you need a drug to get it working properly again. Had I been treated by a competent therapist at the onset of my depression, perhaps its mere kindling would not have turned into a nightmarish psychic bonfire, and I might not have arrived at the point, a decade later, where I needed medication just to be able to get out of bed in the morning.

As it stands, for a few years after I first began taking medication, after leaving Cambridge and coming back to New York, I stayed away from psychotherapy. I saw a psychopharmacologist who was basically a drug pusher with a medical degree, I filled my prescriptions, and believed that that was enough. After Dr. Sterling, I could not imagine ever being able to find a therapist who was good enough. And besides, it seemed that with occasional lapses, drugs really were the answer. But then, as I found myself ruining relationships, alienating employers and other people I worked with, and falling all too frequently into depressive blackouts that would go on for days and would feel as desolate and unyielding as the black wave scares I'd spent much of my pre-Prozac life running from, I realized I needed therapy. Years and years of bad habits, of being attracted to the wrong kinds of men, of responding to every bad mood with impulsive behavior (cheating on my boyfriend or being lax about my work assignments), had turned me into a person who had no idea how to function within the boundaries of the normal, nondepressive world. I needed a good therapist to help me learn to be a grown-up, to show me how to live in a world where the phone company doesn't care that you're too depressed to pay the phone bill, that it turns off your line with complete indifference to such nuances. I needed a psychologist to teach me how to live in a world where, no matter how many people seem to be on Prozac, the vast majority are not, and they've got problems and concerns and interests that are often going to be at odds with my own.

It has taken me so long to learn to live a life where depression is not a constant resort, is not the state I huddle into as surely as a drunk returns to his gin, a junkie goes back to her needle—but I'm starting to get to that place. At age twenty-six, I feel like I am finally going through adolescence.

On April 8, 1994, as I was completing this book, Kurt Cobain shot himself in the head and was found dead in his Seattle home. His suicide was quickly reduced by much of the media into an example of a more general generational malaise gone completely amok, and references were made to "the bullet that shot through a generation." Grunge, the musical style that Nirvana did so much to invent and popularize, was described in *Newsweek* as "what happens when children of divorce get their hands on guitars." Cobain's suicide, despite the extremely private nature of his decision or compulsion to hide himself alone in a room and blow his brains out, quickly came to be seen as greatly symbolic.

There is a part of me that understands why. In the last several years, as so many people have started to fall into some version of a dysthymic category, it has become clear that depression is no longer just a private, psychological matter. It is, in fact, a social problem, and an entire culture of depression has developed around it. One of my favorite examples of this

brand of artistic endeavor was the underground movie hit
Slacker. Made for just $23,000, director Richard Linklater's
debut film showed young people in Austin, Texas, all of them
in school or just out, who preferred to idle away their hours
debating the differences between Smurf culture and Scooby-
Doo culture, living cheaply on the wages of menial jobs that
didn't require a college degree and allowed them plenty of
time to lie in bed, watch TV, and slack around. One character, in a moment of truth, admits he doesn't have a job,
saying, "I may live badly, but at least I don't have to work to
do it." Another film about desperation, *sex, lies and videotape*,
won the Palm d'Or at the Cannes Film Festival, and revolved
around the strained, alienated relationships of four people in
Baton Rouge, Louisiana, centering on a young man so dis-
illusioned with love that he'd replaced actual sex with vid-
eotapes of women describing their sexual experiences and
fantasies. This character wears only black (at one point, his
lawyer buddy tells him he looks like "an undertaker for the
art world"), and his lack of affect became a symbol for many
young people of a hopelessness and battle fatigue that could
make someone stop even trying to make human connections.

But of course, a peak moment in depression culture arrived with the tremendous success of Nirvana, whose hit single "Smells Like Teen Spirit" was a call to apathy. This song
was so delighted with its passivity that its central demand was,
"Here we are now, entertain us." In fact, the band's whole
album, *Nevermind*, seemed to be a long list of the many things
that they *didn't* care about. Of course, rock and roll has had
a long and proud history of songs devoted to the downward
spiral of life, but Nirvana would seem to mark the first time
this kind of punk music delivered both a number-one album
and a number-one single. (To put this in perspective, it took
the Sex Pistols' *Never Mind the Bollocks* album *fifteen* years to
sell a million copies.) Even though *Nevermind* was extremely

poppy and melodious in some ways, it was sufficiently abrasive, cynical and angry that it was never expected to sell very well outside of the alternative-lifestyle circles that had made *Generation X* and *Slacker* into cult hits. When the album did take off, Geffen, the record company behind Nirvana, was caught so far off guard that it didn't have the stock to fill store orders fast enough to meet the demand.

In the meantime, the moody, macabre British new wave bands like the Cure, the Smiths, and Depeche Mode—once considered too depressing for the mainstream—were selling out shows at twenty-thousand seat arenas and finding their largest American followings with suburban mall rats, not the arty intellectuals they were always thought to appeal to. Nine Inch Nails, an industrial noise band from Cleveland, released the appropriately titled album *Pretty Hate Machine* on a small, independent label, and with the help of an absolutely morbid, misanthropic single called "Head Like a Hole," they ended up with a gold record. Jane's Addiction went platinum while advocating heroin abuse, and the Red Hot Chili Peppers were pleasantly surprised when "Under the Bridge," a song about drug withdrawal and suicide attempts, became a number-one single.

Misery-chic achieved a twisted, perverse apotheosis of sorts when the desire to look as gloomy, downtrodden, and nihilistic as Nirvana fans caused designers like Marc Jacobs of Perry Ellis to dispense with haute couture and put dirty flannel shirts and ripped jeans on the Paris runways. Grunge was hailed as the new fashion statement in *Vogue* and made it to the front page of the "Style" section of the *New York Times*. In April 1994, Linda Wells, the editor in chief of *Allure*, wrote that while surveying the pictures of "bone-thin models wearing gloomy, miserable expressions" or looking "anorexic, clinically depressed, or headed for a mental institution," she had to conclude that "something happened to fashion and fashion photography in the past year. It was as if we were all in desperate need of Prozac." Nirvana, whose success had initially been dismissed as a music business anomaly, was actually part of a larger trend.

At the height of Nirvana's popularity, when they managed to both top the charts and smash their instruments on *Saturday Night Live*, I remember thinking that American youth must be really pissed off to have turned something like this into a hit. Jonathan Poneman, one of the owners of Sub Pop Records, an independent Seattle label that first discovered Nirvana, thought the band's success was a sign that the "loser rebellion" was under way. At long last, all of the outcasts, the miserable majority who could never relate to Paula Abdul in the first place, had gone into record stores and demanded to buy music that spoke to them. Trademark Sub Pop T-shirts with the word LOSER printed in caps across the chest became collector's items. Eddie Vedder, the lead singer of a multiplatinum act called Pearl Jam, wore his LOSER T-shirt for several national TV appearances. Then in 1994, another Geffen act, a young man who simply called himself Beck, surprised his label by turning a catchy rap-style folk song called "Loser" into a hit single and a slacker anthem. If being a loser could become cool—and if Nirvana could sell ten million copies of *Nevermind*, have a collection of outtakes and B-sides called *Incesticide* go gold, and watch the album's follow-up, *In Utero*, debut at number one—it was clear that the culture of depression must have been thoroughly entrenched in the mainstream.

So I understand why people might see Kurt Cobain's death as symbolic. Because, after all, they would be perfectly correct to see his life and the music he created in that short time as utterly symbolic. Nirvana's popularity either inaugurated or coincided with some definite and striking cultural moments. No one can or ever should even think to take that away from him or his memory. But by the time he was alone in his garage apartment with a shotgun in his hand with the intent of doing himself in, his actions were far beyond any kind of cultural momentum we can associate with the times. Sylvia Plath killed herself in 1963, before there were slackers and before there were even hippies. She killed herself because she was depressed, the same as Ernest Hemingway, Vince Foster, and so many anonymous others. No one shoots himself in the head because he's had a bad fishing season or because the *Wall Street Journal*'s editorial page says mean things about him. Depression strikes down deep. The fact that depression seems to be "in the air" right now can be both the cause and result of a level of societal malaise that so many feel. But once someone is a clinical case, once someone is in a hospital bed or in a stretcher headed for the morgue, his story is absolutely and completely his own. Every person who has experienced a severe depression has his own sad, awful tale to tell, his own mess to live through. Sadly, Kurt Cobain will never get that far. Every day, I thank God that I did.

July 1986–May 1994

Afterword
(1995)

* * *

By the time the hardcover edition of *Prozac Nation* was published in the autumn of 1994, I thought that I *knew* depression. After about eight years—on and off—of attempting to write this book, partly overlapped with at least a decade of suffering with the disease, it started to seem like the most intimate relationship I'd ever have would be with depression.

But as I began to do readings and interviews after *Prozac Nation*'s publication, and began to receive both warm, inspiring letters and curious, frightening phone calls from the people who had actually read the book, I was humbled and awed by how much I had to learn. I had no idea, in spite of all the statistics, just how many people suffered from depression. I knew the numbers, but I hadn't understood them in human terms, mostly because depression is a very isolating condition. Though organizations like Depressives Anonymous exist to remedy this solitude, they are not nearly as widely subscribed to as Alcoholics Anonymous and other substance-abuse fellowships (in a typical mental health catch-22, the alienating nature of depression tends to keep its sufferers from finding their way to the very support groups that might help them). As such, every depressive is an island.

And I had no idea what a connection I would be able to create between myself and so many similarly pained, pan- icked, and silenced people through publishing this book. I never expected to get more letters in the last several months than I had cumulatively received in the previous twenty- seven years. I never envisioned the number of people who would come to readings, some bringing me CDs, tapes (thanks for all the great Springsteen bootlegs), worry dolls, vitamin pills, herbal remedies, books of Rilke, tubes of ChapStick, even their own diaries. I never imagined how many people would get in touch with me in some way: After all, writers work alone in a room, not quite sure that anyone will ever read their output—at least, this was how I felt— while still hoping against hope that *someone* might. But when they actually do, it always manages to catch you off guard.

Certainly I felt thoroughly unprepared for some of the things people wanted to know after they read *Prozac Nation*: Any time anybody asked me the simplest question—why had I decided to write this book in the first place?—I found myself cobbling together bits of nonsense and trying to improvise a sensible answer. I'd always say something about how I'd writ- ten a first-person account of my experiences with depression for *Mademoiselle* back in 1990, that I'd received a ton of letters, mostly from young women, from all over the country—from places as foreign to me as Wilkes-Barre, PA, and Terre Haute, IN—which led me to believe that this was a worthy topic, one that could have widespread resonance in book form. And I'd go on in that way as if I'd held a bunch of focus groups, and that all the work it took to write *Prozac Nation* was some small and meager response to market forces.

Sometimes, I would also say that I had tried to write other books about very different topics, that I had tried to be a regular journalist, that I had tried to be an arts critic, that I had tried very hard to get away from thinking or feeling depression in all my professional endeavors, but it just kept creeping up, over and over again, like a palimpsest, a text hidden beneath whatever else I was working on that refused to remain submerged. Finally, and, I guess, inevitably, I gave in to the obsessive hold that my experiences with depression seemed to have on me, and decided to just write a whole book, all by itself, about that very subject and nothing else. Get it done and be done with it.

And once I explained to my various interlocutors what I thought might have been my motives for writing *Prozac Nation*, more—and much more—of the real truth would begin to spill out. Because the next question would almost always be, *What on earth makes a woman in her mid-twenties, thus far of no particularly outstanding accomplishment, have the audacity to write a three-hundred page volume about her own life and nothing more, as if anyone else would actually give a shit?*

That was the tough question—and, I think, the *real* question, after the polite precursor—the one that truly made me nervous, because it suggested that I had been presumptuous, and it smacked of accusations of that deadly sin called pride. I hated that. And I hated—for similar reasons—often being introduced or described as "the author of the controversial book," because *Prozac Nation* is, as far as I'm concerned, a memoir with no particular thesis or point, nothing in it championing any cause that could be constructed as "controversial," telling only a small, personal tale of one girl's mental hell. I was mystified—for lack of a better word—by how such a large adjective could so often be connected with what felt to me like my little book. But eventually I had to admit that the contentiousness it sometimes inspired comes down to the simple fact that anyone who is my age, healthy, comfortable, not starving, not dying, not saving the world, not doing much of anything really, would appear to have a great deal of nerve in daring to publish her life story in which she unapologetically asserts that the problems that go on in a place nowhere more momentous than her own head are worth telling the world about.

In effect, if *Prozac Nation* has any particular purpose, it would be to come out and say that clinical depression is a real problem, that it ruins lives, that it ends lives, that it very nearly ended *my* life; that it afflicts many, many people, many very bright and worthy and thoughtful and caring people, people who could probably save the world or at the very least do it some real good, people who are too mired in despair to even begin to unleash the lifespring of potential that they likely have down deep inside. I wanted this book to dare to be completely self-indulgent, unhesitant, and forthright in its telling of what clinical depression feels like: I wanted so very badly to write a book that felt as bad as it feels to feel *this* bad, to feel depressed. I wanted to be completely true to the experience of depression—to the thing itself, and not to the mitigations of translating it. I wanted to portray myself in the midst of this mental crisis precisely as I was: difficult, demanding, impossible, unsatisfiable, self-centered, self-involved, and above all, self-indulgent. As I found myself saying to not a few people who would tell me they found the book angering and annoying to read: Good. Very good: That means I did what I had set out to do. That means you'd felt a frustration and fury reading the book that might even be akin to the sense of futility experienced by most people who try to deal in real life with an actual depressive. Depression is a very narcissistic thing, it's a self-involvement that is so deep and intense that it means the sufferer cannot get out of her own head long enough to see what real good, what genuine loveliness, there is in the world around her.

In my case, the depression created an atmosphere in which I was too stuck inside myself to appreciate the education I was receiving at Harvard, the good friends I was always lucky enough to somehow find, the real love that my mother tried to show me, the real fortune that I had in professional prospects and in a future of good life in general.

I hope that I, in my book, gave a face to what depression really looks like: In many instances, it looks an awful lot like me.

There were other difficulties I ran into in discussing *Prozac Nation*. After all, with the troubles in Bosnia and Rwanda, with the problems that plague inner cities and impoverished backwaters right here in America, what place, on the agenda of national priorities, does a disease of such privilege as depression actually hold?

I really don't know how to answer that. I'm not a public health policy maker, and I don't see any real reason to lobby on behalf of the rights of depressives; I think a great deal of technology (in the form of new medications) and care (in the form of therapy) is quite available to those willing to seek it out, or, in acute cases, to those lucky enough to be dragged to it by their loved ones. But I do think that the prevalence of depression—whether it's clinical or just dysthymic—or something that feels to an awful lot of people like depression, ought to give everyone reason to pause. It has been heartbreaking for me to receive so many letters from teenagers, to see that so many of the readings and signings I do in bookstores are filled with young people, many of whom are on antidepressants, and many of whom have done time in a mental ward or two or more. It is really discouraging to meet thirteen-year-olds who have already been to several psychologists and psychiatrists, who have names of diagnoses that I'm not even all that familiar with—attention deficit disorder, multiple personality disorder, among the more common ones—and who speak without affect about all the treatments they've already been through. It is petrifying to meet parents, many of them single women, who are nervous and scared and want to know what to do about a child who has gone blank, who won't communicate, who hides in his room with earphones and stereo and Metallica albums on, who won't eat or play sports or see friends or take piano lessons anymore.

I can't completely make sense of why so many people are in this condition, but I can certainly see why their plaints, and the ones so shamelessly pounded out in my book, make many people in this country, and made many who commented on my book, feel comfortable declaring it "controversial": After all, what is depression if it isn't the most striking, poignant, psychic challenge to the American Dream? And in that sense, what is my book if not some miserable indictment of the society we live in? Not to sound like some beatnik stuck in the Eisenhower era, but the cry of the depressive is a demand for more and better than what this country has to offer at the apex of privilege. It is a very loud scream that says that happiness is not about status, is not about a two-car garage, is not about money, beachfront property, degrees from fancy schools, membership in prestigious clubs. Were it any of those things, by now I think that *I* would be happy.

But happiness is a difficult thing—it is, as Aristotle posited in *The Nicomachean Ethics*, an activity, it is about good social behavior, about being a solid citizen. Happiness is about community, intimacy, relationships, rootedness, closeness, family, stability, a sense of place, a feeling of love. And in this country, where people move from state to state and city to city so much, where rootlessness is almost a virtue ("anywhere I hang my hat . . . is someone else's home"), where family units regularly implode and leave behind the fragments of divorce, where the long loneliness of life finds its antidote not in a hardy, ancient culture (as it would in Europe), not in some blood-deep tribal rites (as it would in the few still-hale Third World nations) but in our vast repository of pop culture, of consumer goods, of cotton candy for all—in this America, happiness is hard. I don't feel that I'm in any position to make sweeping generalizations about what's wrong with this country, but at least from the small perspective that I've been able to look through in the past year it almost appears as if, around here, everybody *wants* their MTV, everybody's *got* their MTV, and everybody's also got a million other things, lots of other stuff—my God, even kids who live in low-income housing projects can somehow piece together the cash to get their Air Jordans and their VCRs—but happiness just isn't about stuff.

When I finally have to explain my motives for writing this book, it really does come down to wanting to feel less lonely in this lonely feeling, wanting to shed depression's thick, tender, suffocating skin. I wanted to open up and say, *This may not matter to anyone else, but as far as I'm concerned, at times it has felt like I've had Vietnam going on in my own brain.* And I really hoped to reach other people and touch a little bit of their loneliness. When I was in the worst way with my depression, I found solace in music, in Bruce Springsteen, in Joni Mitchell, in Bob Dylan, and in so many other fleeting bits of rock 'n' roll, from Pink Floyd to Flipper to the Joy of Cooking to Janis Joplin. I could never even begin to hope that anything as flat and two-dimensional as words on a page could project outwards and into someone else with the power and alacrity that rock 'n' roll has always been able to enter me, but I wanted to try. It bothered me that rock music, not books, always seemed to be the obvious source of comfort for the young and depressed. Perhaps that was because the great classics of depression literature—*The Catcher in the Rye* and *The Bell Jar*—were written long ago. And the newer books, like William Styron's *Darkness Visible*, always rang false to me, always seemed too polite, too apologetic, too careful—it was often as if Styron was ashamed of what he experienced. And I don't necessarily blame him, he is a great deal older than I am, and depression for him must have seemed a very embarrassing thing indeed, something to hide, to keep inside. But I just wanted to burst. I wanted to write like fever. I wanted to forget all the literary conventions and the hesitation and restraint and sane consideration that I'd always been taught were the hallmarks of good writing. I wanted to write like someone who has been stuck somewhere for so long that by the time she got un-stuck none of the rules mattered anymore. I wanted to write like rock 'n' roll.

And I especially wanted to write *Prozac Nation* for young people. Perhaps it is presumptuous of me to hope that it might give them something to read in their depressive hours that I simply did not have, but I do. And maybe—and this is a really optimistic maybe—somewhere along the way this dour story might give some people some inspiration and even some hope for a better future, for the future that people my age and younger can look forward to building. I met so many bright, amazing, and thoughtful students and recent graduates while I was out touring for *Prozac Nation*, and these encounters have enabled me to picture some grand possibilities of a world that is waiting to be born.

Of course, getting to know some of these rising adults has reminded me that one of the hardest things for parents of depressed or seemingly depressed teenagers to discern is the difference between depression and ordinary adolescence—after all, they have such similar symptoms. It's difficult to know if someone who sleeps until way past lunchtime, thinks shampoo is only used by victims of capitalist corporate oppression, quotes liberally from Anton LeVay (or Herman Hesse or Friedrich Nietzsche), has seen the film version of *The Wall* six times and tries to reenact the nipple-shaving scene at home, thinks Alice Cooper (or Newt Gingrich or Charles Manson) is God Himself, or is into scarification, punk rock, body piercing, or any combination thereof is experiencing a major depressive episode or just being every mother's nightmare. Sometimes it frustrates me to meet the fifteen- and sixteen-year-olds who have read my book, and who already, at such a tender age, have been put on several different medications and can speak with an eerie knowingness about SSRIs and MAO inhibitors and the like; sometimes they almost make me feel glad that I had a few extra years to play my depression out with therapy and other means, because I think it's useful in youth—unless suicide or drug abuse are the alternatives—to have some faith in the mind to cure itself, to not rush to doctors and diagnoses; sometimes I feel lucky that my parents' ineptitude let me believe for a little while that the struggle was just part of growing up. I'm not saying that severe depression in teenagers shouldn't be treated with all available resources and remedies, but I sometimes worry that part of what creates depression in young people is their own, their parents', and the whole world's impatience with allowing the phases of life to run their course. We will very likely soon be living in a society that confuses disease with normal life if the panic and rush to judgment and labeling do not slow down a bit. Somewhere between the unbelievable tardiness that the medical profession was guilty of in administering proper treatment to me and the eagerness with which practitioners prescribe Ritalin for eight-year-old boys and Paxil for fourteen-year-old girls, there is a sane course of action.

Depression, like adolescence, springs at least in part from a feeling of not being quite connected, of being at some in-between stage, of being stuck in the middle, of not quite being able to claim an identity. Imagine *Hamlet* with no end, picture the Hanging Man as the only card in the tarot deck. At twenty-seven, I still feel like an adolescent so very often; I still wonder if I'll ever do the things that grown-ups do— you know, like falling in love, staying in love, having a healthy enough relationship to feel like it could turn itself into a possible home, having a healthy enough credit rating so that I might ever actually be able to buy a home. Thanks to the readers who have responded to this book, I at least feel that there is some use to be found in what I've come to think of as my so-called life. And I owe so much more than I could ever pay for how good that's made me feel.

April 1995
New York City

Acknowledgments

* * *

Without Betsy Lerner, this book quite simply would not have been possible. It's not that it might have come together in a different or lesser form—it's that it would not have happened at all. I know: This project began, and assumed various other guises, back in 1986; over the years, many have tried and none has succeeded—a couple even lost their jobs in the process—to extract the manuscript from me. Only Betsy could have done it. As far as I can tell, she is the best book editor on earth. She's also been a great friend, the big sister I never had, and Job's most likely successor in the patience department. She also happens to be the coolest thirtysomething I've ever met.

The luckiest day of my life was the day I met Mort Janklow, who, as far as I'm concerned, is a crown prince, a swell guy, a brilliant agent, and the master of composing the vituperative-but-still-somehow-encouraging letter (I should frame some of his correspondence.) He is the first person who saw what a mess I was making of my whole career and explained that it didn't have to be that way. Mort is a man who is on your side when he says he's on your side. He's got this great way of telling you everything is going to be just fine, even when it so obviously is not, and then, because he says so, somehow it magically is. How does he do it? I can't thank him enough. It has also been my great good fortune to have Lydia Wills as an agent. Lydia amazes me. She can negotiate these great deals (even with people who barely speak English), offer smart editorial insight and good advice, and still find time at the end of the day just to gossip and be a fellow chick who's a lot of fun. She also has great shoes. But most importantly, her patience and enthusiasm, along with a willingness to take my hysterical phone calls at all hours and even to lend me her apartment to write in when nothing else seemed to be working, meant so much to me.

Houghton Mifflin has been a wonderful publisher, so I must thank John Sterling for taking me into the fold; Jayne Yaffe for being a great copy editor, and for having not one but two copies of the *Physicians' Desk Reference;* Robert Grover for being Betsy's assistant, for being a pal, and for having an unusual concept of how fractions work; Ken Carpenter for being a marketing genius and all-around good guy, the only New Yorker I know who has a camouflage-print video camera; Peter Strupp for headaches yet to come; Christina Coffin for allowing this crash to happen; Becky Saikia-Wilson for production under pressure; Melodie Wertelet for designing this book so beautifully; Debbie Engel for her warmth, interest, and enthusiasm; Hilary Liftin for generously and graciously taking me on late in the game; and the many other people at the company whom I have yet to get to know really, but who have been so kind and helpful already. Janklow and Nesbit has also reaffirmed my faith in the agenting process, so besides Mort and Lydia, I must thank Eric Simonoff, Maria Gallagher, Eileen Godlis, Bennett Ashley, and everybody else over there for making that office the best and most efficient ally any author could ask for. Thanks to Amy Guip for making the cover of this book so very incredible, and to Marion Ettlinger (the coolest fortysomething on earth) for making the girl in the author photo look like someone I'd actually want to be.

According to rabbinical teachings, every time God gets so angry that He finds Himself wanting to blow up the world and put an end to us all, there are thirty-six extremely righteous people roaming the planet who give Him reason to give us another chance. I'm certain that Gail and Stanley Robles are two of them. They are also, most certainly, the coolest of all my friends' parents. They allowed me to stay in their home in sunny Florida so I could get my work done in peace, and they did this without even meeting me first. I still can't figure out what inspired their incredible kindness, but I know they really helped make the world seem like a happier, homier place. Their son, Peter Robles, has also been a great friend, and I thank him forever for hooking me up with his parents. I also thank him for many great meals, great conversations and good times, even if I do feel a need to run out of the room whenever he begins a conversation with something like "The thing about Stravinsky . . ."

In general, if your life is going to be one long emergency, it's a good idea to have good friends. I have been truly blessed in this way. Christine Fasano is a great girl, a loyal friend who has often made me feel comparatively sane—but most importantly, she's been there when I needed her and even when I didn't. She's also had the good sense to earn a living so the rest of us don't have to. Jason Bagdade is an extraordinary roommate, a micromanager to the stars, a provider of *New York Times* crossword puzzles, and my favorite boy on earth. It's a pity we don't want to marry each other, but we just don't. We have disproved the thesis of *When Harry Met Sally*—that men and women simply can't be just friends—over what is starting to seem like eons of living together. My girlfriends over the years have been the glue that kept me together. Sharon Meers, Roberta Feldman, Jody Friedman, Heather Chase, Naomi Shechter, Rachel Brodie: These women are my heroes. There have been other people who've come into my life more recently, many of them have read parts of this book and offered their suggestions, and many have abstained from the process and just been great drinking buddies (and I don't even drink). Here's to the whole sick crew: David Samuels, Elizabeth Acker(wo)man, Mark McGurl, Tom Campbell, Ronnie Drenger, Larissa Macfarquhar, Stefanie Syman, Joe Penachio, Emily Jenkins, and David Lipsky. A special thanks to Betsey Schmidt, who read the manuscript, gave encouragement, and has become a good friend in the process. Andy Lyman, now in the new Europe, which he says is a lot like the old New Jersey, was there when the bank just wasn't. J. C. Weiss was great on copyright detail, better on Wild Turkey duty and a pal to boot.

Nathan Nichols deserved more and better from me. My love and appreciation are with him always, so far beyond anything any paltry words could say.

Bob Gottlieb read a very early draft of this book and offered some very sound advice. He did this on his own time, out of the goodness of his heart, and that really made a difference. I also must thank him for bringing me to *The New Yorker,* and offering me the privilege of having the best job ever. Chip McGrath was hard to get to know at first, but became a very insightful editor, and, I believe, a real friend. Nancy Franklin, a tough broad and a terrific editor, helped improve my writing so very much. Steve Florio, who certainly had many better things to do besides advising overwrought young writers, will always be appreciated for finding the time. Abby McGanney at *Mirabella* and Ralph Novak at *People* have both been true friends and great screening partners over the years. Ed Kosner and Laurie Jones, who at one time were my bosses at *New York,* probably have no idea how much I appreciate the opportunities they gave me. I really do.

There are many people who in a professional and often personal capacity have offered me so much advice and help over the years. Some of them don't even know that I feel the gratitude I do because, sadly, I sometimes have a strange way of showing it. I want these people to know that their care has meant and means a lot: Elaine Pfefferblit, Peter Herbst, Michael Hirschorn, and Jan Miller come particularly to mind.

To Andrea Hedin, M.D., I will be forever grateful. Much appreciation also to Phyllis Zilkha, Ph.D., for therapy that actually works and to Elizabeth Dane, O.M.D., Ph.D., for herbs, acupuncture, and words of wisdom. Jane Goldberg, Ph.D., might be the only landlady on earth to be not just relieved, but truly grateful, to find that her property is still standing at the end of the month, and that the damage done to her antique armoire and the various relics from the Sistine Chapel are nothing that thousands of dollars and a couple of really good restorers in Florence can't repair. But seriously, what good luck it is for me to pay my rent each month (well, more or less) to a psychoanalyst who deals with whatever damage she finds as an indication of some sort of aggression that needs to be worked through in therapy. Jane has also become a good friend, a terrific adviser on boy problems, and a very supportive and generous person whom I still can't believe I hooked up with via a classified apartment listing in the *Village Voice.* Someday I will pay her all that's in arrears. Dolsie Somah is the reason that there is occasionally a pathway to my bedroom amid all the mess; she's also, as far as I can tell, the most kind and virtuous person on earth. Thanks to Sherly

Ip, Irina, and everyone at the Peter Coppola Salon for being as nice to me as they are to Stephanie Seymour, and for understanding that it is just as hard to write when your roots are growing out as it is to pose for the Victoria's Secret catalogue.

Thanks to John Lambros for being such an apt household metaphor.

Thanks to Zap, the most excellent cat on earth, for being such good company.

Thanks to Beat Rodeo, Brendan, and everyone at the Ludlow Street Café for making Monday nights the best way to start the week.

Thanks to Amy Stein, Renata Miller, and everyone at the Writers' Room.

Thanks to Stephen Olson and Susan Litwack for being the first people to encourage me to write, and for making high school bearable. Thanks finally to Bruce Springsteen, Bob Dylan, Joni Mitchell, Lou Reed, and the other great inventors of words and music that made my adolescence, and my depression, somehow possible to survive.

In memoriam:
Richard Whitesell
25 February 1962–13 June 1994
Russell Smith
11 November 1956–16 February 1995
He alone is dead who has been forgotten.